Training With Bodyweight for Strength and Mobility

The content of this book was carefully researched. However, readers should always consult a qualified medical specialist for individual advice before adopting any new exercise program. This book should not be used as an alternative to seeking specialist medical advice.

All information is supplied without liability. Neither the author nor the publisher will be liable for possible disadvantages, injuries, or damages.

Guido Bruscia

TRAINING WITH BODYWEIGHT FOR STRENGTH AND MOBILITY

OVER 70 FUNCTIONAL TRAINING EXERCISES TO BUILD MUSCLE AND STAY LIMBER

The Ultimate Functional Training Series, Volume I

Meyer & Meyer Sport

Original title: *Allenamento Funzionale – Manuale scientifico,*
© Guido Bruscia, 2013 Elika Srl Editrice via Fossalta 3895-47522 Cesena

Translation: AAA Translation, www.aaatranslation.com

British Library Cataloguing in Publication Data
A catalogue record for this book is available from the British Library

Training With Bodyweight for Strength and Mobility
Maidenhead: Meyer & Meyer Sport (UK) Ltd., 2025
ISBN: 978-1-78255-273-4

© 2025 by Meyer & Meyer Sport (UK) Ltd.
Aachen, Auckland, Beirut, Cairo, Cape Town, Dubai, Hägendorf, Hongkong, Indianapolis,
Manila, New Dehli, Singapore, Sydney, Tehran, Vienna

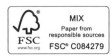 Member of the World Sport Publishers' Association (WSPA), www.w-s-p-a.org

Printed by Print Consult GmbH, Munich, Germany
Printed in Slovakia

CREDITS
Cover design: Kristina Ehrhardt, Anja Elsen
Cover photos: © Guido Bruscia and Thinkstock/iStock
Photos: Chapter images on p. 18, 19 32, 33, 35, 44, 45, 64, 80, 91, 111: Shutterstock (www.shutterstock.com)
Chapter graphics: © Thinkstock/iStock
The rights to all photo remain with the publish
Layout: Kristina Ehrhardt, Anja Elsen
Typesetting: www.satzstudio-hilger.de
Copyediting: Elizabeth Evans

ISBN: 978-1-78255-273-4
E-Mail: info@m-m-sports.com
www.thesportspublisher.com

CONTENTS

ACKNOWLEDGMENTS...

To my family, for never failing to embrace me.

To Ester, my partner and "muse", for our life together.

To my grandmother Sara, 106 years old, still functional today.

To Ernesto Rossi and Sabrina Parrello (and their children Ettore and Giovanni), for their great, true and unconditional friendship.

...AND THANKS

This book was born many years ago and is the work of the author and of all those who have been for him, even if unaware of it, a source of inspiration and ideas:

Emilio They (a friend and master never mourned enough), Marco Neri, Steve Cotter, Michael Boyle, Robert Dos Remedios, Alwin Cosgrove, Martin Rooney, Stuart McGill, Todd Durkin, Josh Henkin, Michol Dalcourt, Gray Cook, Marc Lebert, and many others who, for reasons of space (and memory!), I cannot mention.

Thank you also to all the friends, students, and colleagues who follow me with affection and respect.

Here, too, I can do justice to only a few of them:

Eda Maistrelli, Roberto Braghiroli, Claudio Arena, Emanuele Gollinucci, Roberto Cappelletti, my students at the Hamazon courses in Piombino and Castiglione della Pescaia, Bruno and Serena and the Mensana gym staff in Grosseto, Marco Giannoni and the Palestra Azzurra gym staff in Follonica, Mirko, and Cesare and the Living Club gym staff in Piombino.

Thanks also to the companies that help me with my work:

Elika Editrice

FitnessBest Innovation

Libertas

Ledraplastic

Tecnocomponent

Technogym

Newvitality

Superdry

Xconcept

Vibram Fivefingers

Vistawell

FOREWORD

Ever since humankind appeared on earth, people have always interacted with the environment in their own way.

Civilization has brought infinite advantages to the life of human beings but has also made them weaker and more imperceptive. The senses of smell, hearing and touch, proprioception, and the various organic capacities have all undergone modifications in the course of evolution from our ancestors to the present day. The result is that, while on the one hand we live in heated homes, on the other, a gust of wind is enough to send us to bed with a fever (Marlo Morgan, *E venne chiamata due cuori*).

Galen, one of the fathers of medicine (131-201 AD), wrote in his work *De sanitate tuenda:*

"...This is what I consider as physical exercise or gymnastics, a term connected with the gymnasium, where people go to anoint themselves, enjoy a massage, engage in wrestling, discus throwing or other sporting activities."

More than one thousand years after that, Mercurial recommended discus throwing, rope climbing, race walking, mountain climbing, and long jump as the activities that had the most benefits. People used to train with more or less rudimentary weights: medicine balls, dumbbells, rocks, the trapeze, ropes and still rings.

An athlete had to be strong, fast, and resilient.

Today, the immense popularity of gyms has produced centers which are extremely well-equipped, sophisticated, and multifunctional. Often, fitness centers imitate outdoor activities with much theatrical effect; they have free-climbing walls meant to resemble jagged, rocky cliffs, water courses and machines that mimic walking, running, and cycling outdoors. And yet, from many quarters, we see signs of a trend in the opposite direction: woodland programs, treetop walks in the woods, life-trails in parks, and a return to body-weight exercises, in which the body is the main training tool. The growing popularity of functional training is a sign that something is changing.

Worn down by the stress of urban life, people are returning to their origins; they are feeling the need for a stroll, a run, a different kind of muscular workout unconstrained by machines or showy equipment. They are looking for woods or meadows.

Nature all around, and, overhead, the sky as the only limit.

INTRODUCTION

When we talk about education, we refer to a system of knowledge which involves different fields of learning and is constantly evolving.

Gym activity requires the knowledge of physiology, anatomy, and biomechanics. Knowledge of nutrition and supplements also has proven to have an influence on sports performance and on results, and not just in terms of achievements. Also, in recent years, several studies have overturned many ideas and misconceptions connected with the world of sports.

Knowledge is an imperfect journey, full of trial and error. To these facts we have to add, of course, exercise practice, an empirical science which is by no means a given. Contrary to most beliefs, practice does not make us perfect: It is perfect practice that makes us perfect. The objective of education is to create professionalism, a word which, today like never before, plays a fundamental role in a coach's assessment. A professional is someone who provides a unique performance. Let's not forget this.

WARNING

This textbook has been written with the average fitness enthusiast in mind.

For this reason, I have glossed over issues which aren't strictly germane to the theme and sacrificed the purely technical definition of several concepts in favor of a more direct, straightforward language.

Medicalese doesn't help in assimilating concepts.

RESOLUTIONS

In 2004, at a personal trainers convention, I lectured on:

"Functional training for the lower limbs: A new perspective." In subsequent years, I studied the functional subject in depth, comparing my findings with those of several gurus in the USA, Spain, Switzerland, Germany, Slovenia, and Italy.

Functional training changes your life. Not your sporting life, which is focused on the search for optimal performance or, accordingly, for hypertrophy and super-toned bodies. Functional training simply makes people feel better, making them more active, stronger, tougher. In a few weeks, you will notice that your health is changing and that your physical efficiency and the well-being you are enjoying today have reached new heights. All this is the result of an optimization of factors which contribute to building a new body. It will not just be a matter of being more toned; there will be the awareness of feeling efficient for the first time.

Your body is like a custom-made outfit: It is the best place to live in.

All you have to do is try.

PART I – THEORY

1

THE LOCOMOTOR APPARATUS

1.1   PRESENTATION

Every time we think about a sporting activity, we associate it with the concept of *motion*.

This process is so widespread and natural that we don't think about its underlying reason *why*. During courses, students who are interested in and passionate about training sometimes ask me why it is necessary to know stuff that has no apparent connection with a horizontal bench or a squat.

The answer is that gymnastics, in its broadest sense, is an empirical science; it stands apart from scientific bases which interact constantly with sporting exercise in gyms or outdoors. For this reason, you will often find not only various definitions, but also examples which refer back to practice.

The locomotor apparatus is the structure that allows a person to move in relation to space and the outside world. For practical purposes, it is subdivided into an active part and a passive part. The active part is made up of muscles, tendons, and ligaments. The inactive part is composed of bones and joints. Each is briefly discussed in the following sections.

1.1.1   The active part of the locomotor apparatus: Muscles, tendons, and ligaments

MUSCLES

The term *muscle*, from the Latin *musculus* (from *mus*, rat, because some movements are reminiscent of a rat darting about), indicates an organ made of biological tissue with the ability to contract.

The muscles are subdivided into:

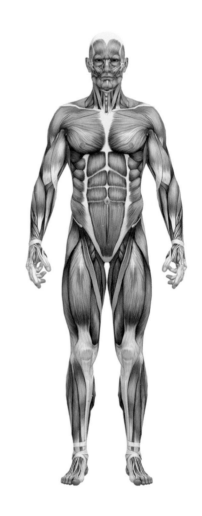

- Smooth, or involuntary, muscles
  Commanded by the autonomic nervous system, they encase the walls of several organs and corporeal systems, enabling or improving their functionality with their contraction.

- Striated skeletal, or voluntary, muscles
  Commanded by the central nervous system, they encase the skeleton, and, by their contraction (shortening), they determine the bone levers' movement.

A peculiar type of striated muscle is the myocardium, which is commanded by the autonomic nervous system.

TENDONS

Tendons are bands of connective tissue with poor elasticity, and their function is to anchor the muscles to the bones. Their role is to transmit tension from muscles to the bone levers, thus allowing their movement.

LIGAMENTS

Ligaments are sheaves of connective tissue with varying percentages of collagen fibers that link bones at the joints. The ligaments' purpose is to limit articular movement which would risk creating lesions were it to continue. For example, the knee's collateral medial and lateral ligaments support the anterior and posterior cruciate ligaments in limiting the articulation's intra- and extrarotation movements in order to avoid lesions to the knee itself.

1.1.2   The passive part of the locomotor apparatus: Bones and joints

BONES

Bones are specialized tissues with great mechanical resistance. They are divided into:

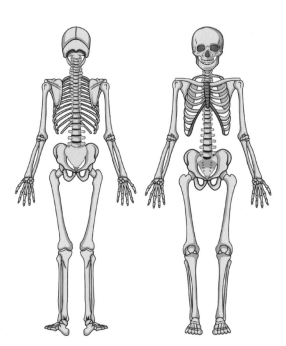

- Long bones (humerus, femur, tibia, radius): These are composed of an elongated body known as *diaphysis* and by terminal extremities known as *epiphysis*; they determine raw movements, which are characterized by wide articular excursions.
- Short bones (vertebrae): They have a similar diameter in all three spatial dimensions.
- Irregular bones (facial bones, the patella): These bones are characterized by variable dimensions and shape.
- Flat bones (pelvis, sternum, skull): Their function is protecting internal organs.

Don't be misled by bone tissue in the passive part of the locomotor apparatus: The bone is a highly active and dynamic tissue. In fact, from birth, the bone undergoes a remodeling process, involving the change and overlap of catabolic and anabolic phases. The catabolic phases are stimulated by micro organelles called *osteoclasts*, and the anabolic phases are activated by other specialized cells called *osteoblasts*. The piezoelectric effect gives the input for an increased bone tissue synthesis activity.

What does it involve? During motor activity, bone segment compression generates an electric depolarization of the bone membrane at the load points. This creates a greater localized need for the reconstructive osteoblasts. This explains why weight training, as demonstrated by several studies, has turned out to be an excellent remedy to contrast osteoporosis.

JOINTS

Joints are the junction hubs between two or more bone segments around which bones rotate.

According to their configuration and degree of mobility, joints can be classified as follows:

- **Synarthroses:** These are fixed, fibrous joints with little or no possibility of movement.
- **Amphiarthroses:** These joints are semi-mobile; they are often cartilaginous (e.g., vertebrae).
- **Diarthroses:** These are the mobile, synovial joints capable of a greater degree of movement. In terms of movement range, the most significant are the enarthroses (e.g., shoulder and hip), with spherical-shaped, multi-axial articular surfaces.

1.2   MUSCLE ACTION

For clarity, I have simplified the different muscular actions, adding the technical definition in parentheses.

- **Flexion:** When two bone segments move closer to each other (the moving part draws away from the horizontal plane). Example: brachial biceps, femoral biceps
- **Extension:** When two bone segments move away from each other (the moving part draws nearer to the horizontal plane). Example: brachial triceps, femoral quadriceps
- **Adduction:** When a bone segment draws closer to the median sagittal line (the moving part draws closer to the sagittal plane). Example: thigh adductors group
- **Abduction:** When a bone segment draws away from the median sagittal line (the moving plane draws away from the median sagittal plane). Examples: gluteus minimus and gluteus medius, high tensor fascia, deltoid
- **Torsion:** Movement of the trunk around the vertical axis.
- **Rotation:** Movement of a limb on its longitudinal axis.
- **Intrarotation:** Rotation of a bone segment in the medial direction, in other words, toward the inside (movement toward the anterior frontal plane).
- **Extrarotation:** Rotation of a bone segment in the lateral direction, in other words, toward the outside (movement toward the posterior frontal plane).

Each muscle performs several movements, which must be differentiated in order to better define exercises and their completion. For example, flexion and extension take place when the limbs aren't bearing weight. Bending, however, takes place when the limbs are bearing weight, as when completing a push-up. We may therefore notice that what is commonly referred to as flexing the arms is defined more correctly as bending the arms.

1.3   ROLE OF THE INDIVIDUAL MUSCLES

Based on the role they play in movement, we may differentiate muscles as:

- **Agonist muscles:** They play the main role in a specific action. Example: pectoral muscles in the horizontal bench press.
- **Antagonist muscles:** In the same action, they play an opposite role to the agonist muscles. Example: the trapezius muscle in the horizontal bench press.
- *Synergistic muscles* (from the Greek *sun-ergo*, "working together"): They help and support the agonist muscles. Examples: the triceps and anterior deltoid muscles in the horizontal bench press.
- *Neutralizing muscles* (stabilizers): They stabilize a bone segment, allowing other muscles to execute a certain action.
- *Fixator muscles:* They act as stabilizers, but they that is not their only role. They block a segment in the position that is appropriate to a movement or an action. Examples: pectoralis and latissimus dorsi muscles in parallel bars exercises.

1.4   ARTICULAR FEATURES OF MUSCLES

In gyms, muscle articulation is mostly disregarded, if not completely ignored.

Yet muscle articulation is of fundamental importance in understanding how to teach various exercise methods. Muscle articulation is defined as:

- **monoarticular,** those muscles that control only one joint and are inserted on bone levers that are paired by one joint only; and
- **bi- or multiarticular,** those muscles that cross over two or more joints.

In order to understand the importance of this distinction, let me remind you that when a muscle is biarticular, it should be stimulated with biarticular movements in order to be fully trained.

The most common example is that of the biceps brachii. Though it is a biarticular muscle, the biceps brachii is usually trained with monoarticular movements—the upper arm is kept steady against the trunk while only the forearm moves. To be clear, the monoarticular movement in this case isn't wrong, but it is nevertheless incomplete.

1.5   MUSCULAR TISSUE FEATURES

The features of muscular tissue are the following:

- **Contractility:** a muscle's ability to shorten.
- **Extensibility:** a muscle's ability to lengthen.
- **Elasticity:** the muscle tissue's ability to return to the initial length from a stretching position (the time factor needs to be evaluated, too).
- **Tonicity:** a very low-intensity electrical message which is always present within the muscle, even when at rest.

A common mistake is assuming that stretching helps only to elongate the muscle. In reality, there are many more effects of stretching:

- Extensibility
- Elasticity
- Articular flexibility
- Elongation of the connective tissue

For many years now, the concept of analytic stretching, in other words, stretching a single muscle or articular segment, has been surpassed in favor of systemic stretching, which involves longer muscular and articular chains.

More accurately, today we talk about mobilization, with reference to

- the joints, where muscles connect; and
- the connective tissue which covers the muscles and is less extensible than the joints; this means that when you talk about stretching a muscle, actually the range of the stretch is deeply influenced by the elasticity of the tissue that covers it.

1.6   ELEMENTS OF BIOMECHANICS: LEVERS

Biomechanics is the science that studies the law of mechanical actions in living systems.

Sports biomechanics studies a human being's movement within the process of physical exercise.

The study of biomechanics is essential when approaching any motor or sporting activity in order to identify

- the body's structure and motor functions; and
- the specific technique of the sport being studied.

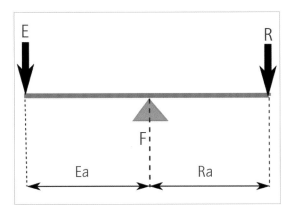

Lever in balance

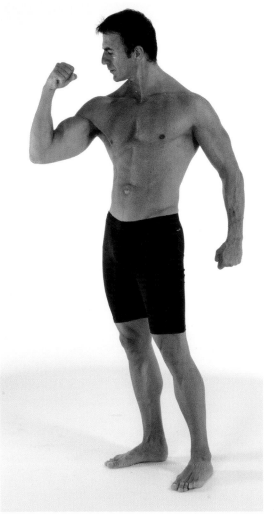

A *lever* is a simple machine consisting of a rigid segment tied to a fixed point called a fulcrum (F), upon which two forces of equal strength but opposite direction are applied, called effort (E) and resistance (R).

The distance from the fulcrum to the point where resistance is applied is called the resistance arm (Ra); the distance from the fulcrum to the point where effort is applied is called the effort arm (Ea).

A lever is in balance when the resistance and effort arms are equal.

A lever is disadvantageous when the resistance arm is greater than the effort arm.

A lever is advantageous when the effort arm is greater than the resistance arm.

If we think about it, we realize that our skeletal system is a set of levers:

- Bones are the rigid segments.
- The fulcrum consists of the various joints that are involved.
- Resistance consists of the weight (load) we apply to the various levers.
- Effort consists of the muscles which contrast the weight's action.

The application point of resistance (i.e., where the resistance arm departs from) is the point of contact between the weight and the locomotor apparatus. The application point of effort (i.e., where the effort arm departs from) is where the muscle inserts into the bone segment. There are three types of levers in the human body, separated according to the distribution of the effort and resistance forces and the fulcrum around which the various bone segments hinge:

Type 1: Inter-fulcrum lever

The fulcrum is always positioned between effort and resistance. As we saw, a lever is advantageous, disadvantageous, or in balance according to whether the effort arm is greater than, smaller than, or equal to the resistance arm.

Example: a pair of scissors, a 45-degree calf exercise at the press machine.

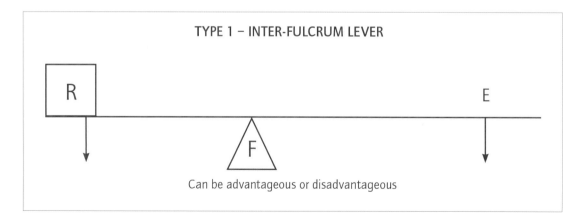

TYPE 1 – INTER-FULCRUM LEVER

R   E

F

Can be advantageous or disadvantageous

Type 2: Inter-resistance lever

From its name we can deduce that resistance will always be positioned between the fulcrum and effort. The effort arm, therefore, is always greater than the resistance arm. The lever is always advantageous.

Example: nutcracker, standing calf raise exercise.

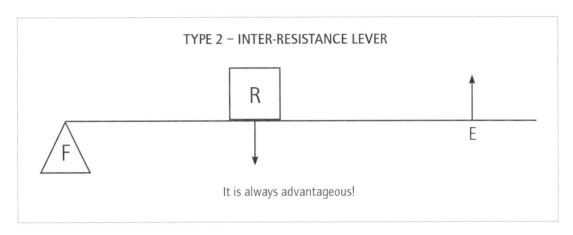

Type 3: Inter-effort lever

The same logic applies: Effort will always be located between fulcrum and resistance. The resistance arm is always greater than the effort arm. The lever is disadvantageous.

Example: tweezers, biceps.

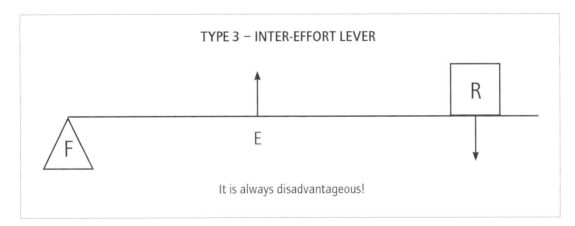

1.6.1   Thoughts on organic levers

The majority of organic levers, at least when it comes to long bones (i.e., great locomotion), are type 3. Our body has opted for a predominance of disadvantageous levers. Why? Because this type of lever, though disadvantageous in terms of strength, allows wider movements and greater articular excursions and at high speeds. In practical terms, the evolutionary choice has been toward greater speed. (Let's keep these features in mind.

ENERGY SYSTEMS

2.1   PRESENTATION

Life on Earth has evolved along the energy road, consuming energy economically and obtaining it easily. All living organisms now extinct (not because of human intervention) were inefficient energy systems and, as such, extremely wasteful. Living, making the body function, or performing any action requires energy. We can define *energy* as the ability to carry out a task. Specifically, a muscle is a chemodynamic machine; in other words, it functions through chemical reactions.

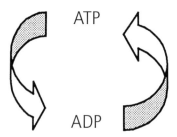

In order to convey a concept, it is useful to use imagery, visualizing the concept in pictures. To simplify the following chemical reaction, I will use imagery. Imagine a car. The model is called Man. Its fuel is adenosine triphosphate, or simply ATP. The human machine's universal fuel (its gasoline) is a molecule possessed of a high degree of chemical energy.

Our cells burn ATP continuously, and they are always synthesizing new ATP to obtain a supply of energy.

The gasoline's combustion in the car, Man, comes from the following reaction:

$$ATP \rightarrow ATPase \rightarrow ADP + P + Energy$$
$$Energy = (7.3 \text{ kcal}/\text{mole})$$

ATP breaks down into adenosine diphosphate, and this reaction produces energy.

The adenosine triphosphatase enzyme catalyzes the reaction (enzymes are substances which catalyze—they influence the speed of biochemical reactions, increasing or decreasing).

The amount of ATP present within cells allows them to work for a few seconds only. So how do they continue to work over time? They activate makeshift energy systems, with the objective of producing ATP (energy) according to the intensity and duration of the activity required. Intensity and duration cannot go hand in hand; they are two inversely proportional parameters. The more intensity (i.e., energy supply) required during an activity, the shorter the activity will be. Conversely, a lower intensity will allow a longer workout. Think about sprinting: You can run 100 m [109 yd] very fast, but you can't keep up the same speed to run, for example, 3,000 m [3,280 yd].

2.2 ANAEROBIC ALACTACID (CREATINE PHOSPHATE) SYSTEM

Let's imagine:

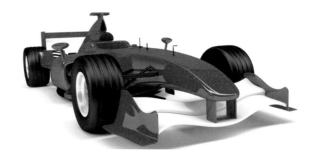

Car: Man
Model: Formula 1
Fuel: ATP + CP

This system is used when an immediate supply of energy is needed for a very high-intensity but short-duration workout: 0-20 min (optimized at around 13 min).

What does the name tell us?

Anaerobic means there is no presence of oxygen; *alactacid* means that no lactic acid is produced.

We use a process called *phosphorylation:* The energy level of a substance is increased by binding it to a phosphoric group.

How is the energy supplied? Let's review the basic reaction:

$$ATP \rightarrow ATPase \rightarrow ADP + P + Energy$$

In this reaction, ATP breaks down into ADP. At this stage, ATP gets recharged by creatine phosphate (CP). CP doesn't supply energy directly, but it supports ADP, retransforming it into ATP, allowing the reaction to continue.

$$ADP + CP \rightarrow cpkase \rightarrow C + ATP$$
(Loehmann's mono-enzyme reaction)

The concentration of CP in the muscle is four to six times higher compared to that of ATP; this allows the energy supply to last a little longer compared to using ATP only.

Examples of sporting activities requiring CP for energy: 60-100 m [65.6-109 yd] sprint, long jump, high jump, strength training

2.3   ANAEROBIC LACTACID SYSTEM

Let's imagine:

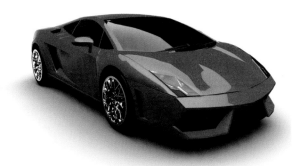

Car: Man
Model: Turbo-diesel sedan
Fuel: Glycogen/ATP

This system is used in performances that require a high energy supply for a medium-short duration. Let's analyze the name again. *Anaerobic* means in the absence of oxygen; *lactacid* means that there is lactic acid, or lactate, production. The ATP molecules are stored inside the muscles and the liver in the form of a complex sugar, an animal polysaccharide: glycogen (you can imagine diesel fuel). ATP is produced when glycogen breaks down into glucose, producing pyruvic acid and, subsequently, lactic acid.

This energy supply process is fast; it allows a high- to medium-intensity workout between 20 sec and 2 min (optimized around 30-40 sec).

The longer time required for the supply of energy compared to the anaerobic alactacid system is due to the 10 chemical reactions that lead to the breakdown of the molecules mentioned above.

Energy comes from the muscular glycogen and the hepatic glucose, according to the following steps:

GLUCOSE
↓
2 ATP
↓
PYRUVIC ACID
↓
LACTIC ACID

When one glucose molecule breaks down into pyruvic acid, two ATP molecules are formed.

This process is also known as *anaerobic glycolysis*.

This being a high-intensity activity with low utilization of oxygen, a highly acidic environment forms inside the muscles. Pyruvic acid binds to two excess H+ ions, producing lactic acid.

$$ADP + P + glucose \ddot{} \ ATP + lactic\ acid$$

When the lactate build-up becomes excessively high, the muscle's contractile capacity is inhibited (hypoxia).

What is the fate of lactic acid? Once the exercise is finished, it is partly used as fuel but it is chiefly re-converted into pyruvic acid and re-stocked in the muscles as muscular and hepatic glycogen (Cori's cycle).

Lactic acid isn't the cause for post-training pains!

2.4 AEROBIC SYSTEM (AEROBIC GLYCOLYSIS OR OXIDATIVE PHOSPHORYLATION IN MITOCHONDRIA)

Let's imagine:

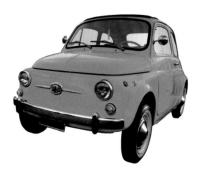

Car: Man
Model: MPV car
Fuel: Macronutrients/ATP

This system is used for all activities ranging from very low to medium intensity, lasting from a few minutes to some hours. Let's take a closer look.

Aerobic means the presence of oxygen is required.

Beyond the 2-min mark, only the presence of oxygen still allows glucose transformation; if the activity lasts longer than this, the system begins to activate processes which use stored fat as fuel. Compared to carbohydrates, lipids have a more unfavorable ratio between hydrogen and oxygen, and this explains the need to capture oxygen from outside to metabolize them. Proteins, too, provide energy within this system but in a lower percentage (3-5%).The process, also called *oxidative phosphorylation*, takes place within mitochondria, the cell's miniature power stations. The start is similar to the anaerobic lactacid system:

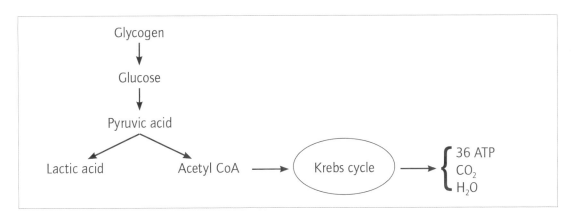

Because this is a reduced-intensity activity, pyruvic acid is transformed into acetyl-coenzyme A and transferred to the mitochondria, entering the Krebs cycle. The latter is like a metabolic furnace inside which the glucose molecule is completely broken down, generating 36 ATP, carbon dioxide, and water molecules.

In order to produce ATP, the aerobic system needs hydrogen. This is supplied by the Krebs cycle, exploiting oxidation (i.e., the removal of hydrogen) of food-derived compounds. Hydrogen is then transported to the respiratory chain via NAD (nicotinamide-nucleotide) and FAD (flavin adenine dinucleotide) up to the final receptor, oxygen, generating water.

Summarizing, the aerobic system is the result of two events:

1. Substrata breakdown, with production of hydrogen and carbon dioxide (Krebs cycle).
2. Hydrogen transportation to the respiratory chain, forming water.

2.5 ENERGY SYSTEM INTERACTIONS

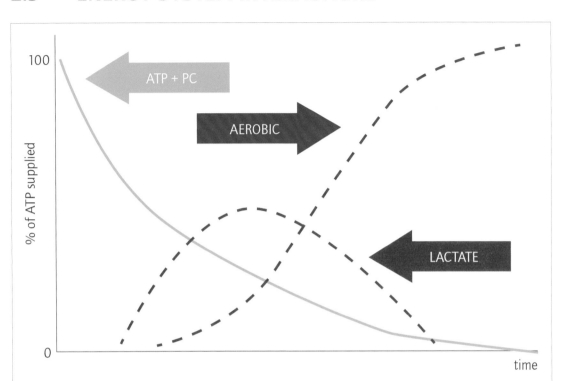

It is important to understand how the three energy systems cooperate.

The basic mechanism used by our body is the aerobic system. All the activities in our normal daily life take place at a low intensity and do not require a high amount of energy. This means that the aerobic system can comfortably provide the energy for all our daily activities. Whenever more intense efforts beyond the aerobic system's capacity are needed, the anaerobic systems work together with the aerobic system.

Note that in supplying energy, the three energy systems do not alternate like a relay. So when the synthesized ATP is active, it does not pass the baton to the anaerobic alactacid system, which in turn does not pass it to the anaerobic lactacid one. Instead, the three systems work together in parallel but also in different percentages, according to the type of effort, its duration, and the related demand for energy.

2.6   VO$_2$MAX AND THE ANAEROBIC THRESHOLD

The concepts connected to the terms *VO$_2$max, anaerobic threshold,* and *oxygen debt* are important.

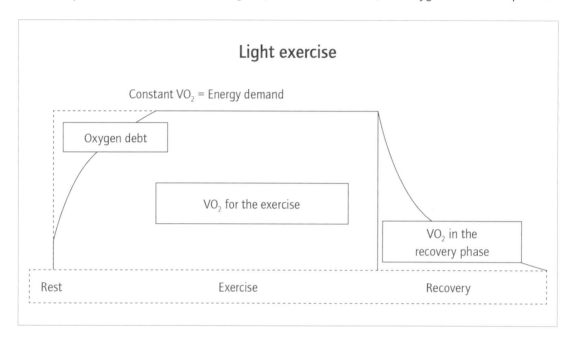

VO$_2$max, or maximum aerobic power, is in practical terms the organism's maximum capacity for synthesizing ATP using aerobics exclusively. It has actually been observed that this figure is more the result of a theoretical calculation than something reproducible in a lab or, even harder, in real life. An athlete is capable of maintaining an effort equal to VO$_2$max for no more than 10 min. Why? Besides a long list of factors—the majority of them genetic—the fact remains that at the experimental level it has been observed that well before reaching this limit the body begins to produce lactic acid. For this reason, at least in fitness training, the concept of anaerobic threshold has become increasingly important.

The **anaerobic threshold** is the maximum level of physical effort the organism can sustain without accumulating lactate in the blood. Above that heart rate the organism begins accumulating lactic acid because it cannot dispose of it as fast as it can produce it. The outcome is the fast onset of fatigue.

2.7   OXYGEN DEBT AND EPOC

Oxygen debt is the increased uptake of oxygen needed to remove excess lactic acid that is created by the increased synthesis of ATP which results from anaerobic physical exercise. What does this mean? We have seen that when you start a motor activity, there is an increase in the body's energy requirements. At the outset, the aerobic system isn't immediately available unless the activity is at a very low intensity.

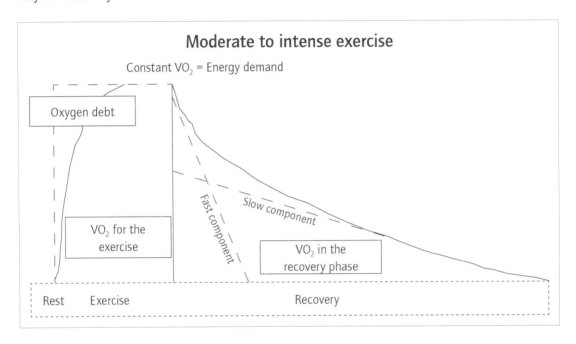

The body, therefore, requires help from the anaerobic systems, increasing the oxygen debt. The greater the intensity of the activity, the larger the debt. As soon as the effort is over, the body pays its debt by increasing oxygen uptake from the outside in order to restore phosphates and remove the lactic acid produced.

Dash or sprint for 20-30 sec. Now stop. What are you doing? You're panting. Your trunk leans forward, and your hands are on your knees. In order to increase your thoracic cavity's capacity, you inhale as much oxygen as possible from the air around you. This is the increased oxygen uptake.

Any exercise which involves the development of power above VO₂max is defined as *supramaximal*.

An oxygen debt can also be incurred as a result of a supramaximal load imposed on muscles; the oxidative machine intervenes in this case, too, at the end of the performance. However, in the ensuing recovery phase, the oxygen uptake exceeds the volume of the deficit. It's as though you're paying your debt with interest.

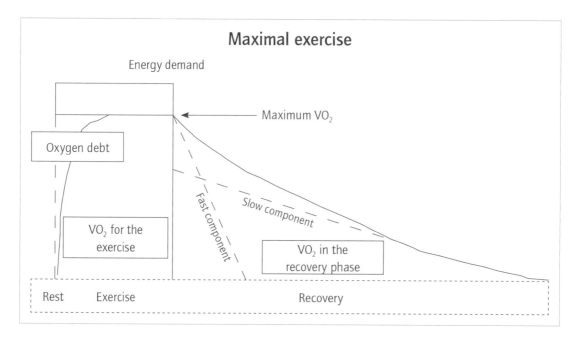

Margaria[1], R. (1938) has shown how the O_2 consumption curve during recovery can be split into four components:

1. **Constant component:** it depends on the subject's metabolism at rest.
2. **Fast component:** payment of the debt's alactacid fraction at a decreasing rate; lactate halves every 30 sec.
3. **Slow component:** payment of the lactacid debt at a slowly decreasing rate because of the energy cost of the renewed glycogen synthesis originating from lactic acid.
4. **Slow, long-lasting component:** attributed to the stimulus effect of the exercise on the metabolism at rest.

---

1 Margaria R. (1938). Sulla fisiologia e specialmente sul consumo energetico della marcia e della corsa a varia velocità ed inclinazione del terreno, in *Atti Accademia Nazionale dei Lincei* 7, 299-368.

With regards to this, studies show how the more intense a training session is, the higher the metabolism remains for a longer period of time in order to compensate the oxygen debt.

Recently, the concept of oxygen debt has been included in the wider concept of EPOC (excess post-exercise oxygen consumption). EPOC includes not just the oxygen debt but also the domino-effect adaptations which depend on it:

- Payment of the alactacid debt.
- Payment of the lactacid debt.
- Increased body temperature.
- Thermogenic effect caused by catecholamines.
- Renewed lactate synthesis.
- Renewed phosphagen synthesis.
- Lactate and blood oxygenation.
- High cardiac frequency.

CHAPTER

3

MUSCULAR CONTRACTION

3.1   PRESENTATION

We have seen in the preceding chapters a presentation of the locomotor apparatus and of the energy systems through which the body acquires energy for movement.

Let's now focus our attention on the muscles, specifically on the processes which lead to muscular contraction and on the phenomena that result.

Let's introduce the main players:

1.   The central nervous system (CNS). It consists of the brain, the cerebellum, and the spinal cord. From here voluntary muscular contraction originates through a nerve impulse.

2.   The drive units. They consist of a body called *motor neuron*, an electric cable, the axon (including an insulating substance, the myelin sheath), and the muscular fibers stemming from it. The drive units' task is to carry the nerve impulse from the CNS to the muscle. The movement input reaches the muscle from the drive unit via a neurotransmitter (i.e., a substance which transmits a nerve impulse, called acetylcholine [Ach]).

3. The muscles. Each muscle is composed of a muscle belly surrounded by a sheath of connective tissue called *epimysium*.

■ *Muscular fibers.* Inside the muscle there are groups of fibers bundled together in primary sheaths, or fascicles, encased by the perimysium. The primary sheaths are formed by muscular fibers encased by the epimysium; muscular fibers are in turn made of myofibrils, sheathed by the endomysium.

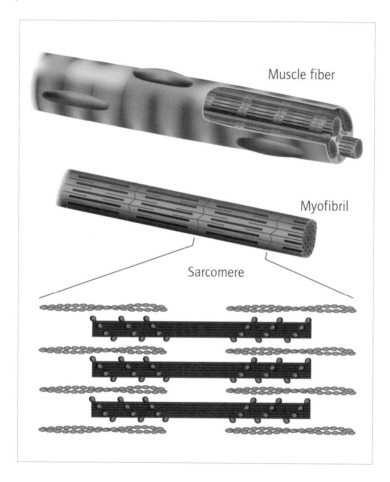

3.2   MUSCULAR CONTRACTION

Viewed through an electron microscope, myofibrils appear as long filaments divided up into compartments by darker strips. Myofibrils can be compared with a train. The single cars, segmented by the Z lines, are called sarcomeres, and they constitute the cell's essential contractile unit. Inside each car (sarcomere) are two main

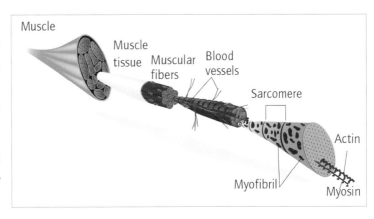

Skeletal muscle structure.

regulatory proteins that partial overlap: actin (which is thinner) and myosin (larger, shaped like an oar or a golf club). We also find two other regulatory proteins, troponin and tropomyosin, interposed between the actin and myosin.

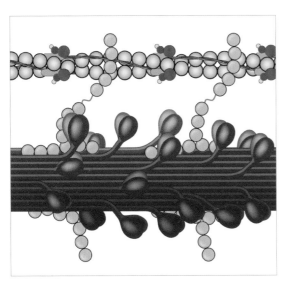

Actin and myosin.

Voluntary muscular contraction originates from the brain, goes through the cerebellum (movement is intermediary, making it fluid and coordinated), and reaches the spinal cord. From the spinal cord, the drive units incite the release of calcium ions from small cisterns called T-shaped tubules by releasing acetylcholine. The calcium ions bind with tropomyosin and troponin, canceling their inhibiting effect on actin and myosin. At this stage, the two main regulatory proteins come into contact. In the presence of ATP, the myosin heads attach to actin, pulling it and making it slide above them.

This sliding process is applied to every sarcomere inside the muscle and leads to its shortening or contraction (Huxley's myofilament sliding theory).

3.3   TYPES OF MUSCLE FIBERS

There exist two main types of muscular fibers, both possessing very different chemical and physical features.

- **Type I fibers,** or red fibers, or slow-twitch fibers.
  They are small and rich in mitochondria. They produce small tensions but are endowed with significant endurance.

- **Type II fibers,** or white fibers, or fast-twitch fibers.
  They are larger and produce high tensions but only for a short time. They hypertrophy very easily and are divided in two subgroups: type IIx and type IIa.

1. *Type IIx fibers* are known as pure white fibers and also as fast glycotic, with very few mitochondria, high tensile capacity and very limited endurance.
2. *Type IIa fibers,* or fast oxidative glycotic are also called intermediate fibers, since they share both some of the red and white fibers' characteristics: a good percentage of mitochondria, fine tensile capacity, and moderate endurance.

The percentage of fibers which innervate a specific muscle points to the type of training needed for it as well. For example, if hypertrophy is the objective, a muscle with a high percentage of white fibers will need to be trained with high weight loads, few repetitions, maximal or submaximal tensions, and long recovery periods. However, a muscle with a high percentage of red fibers will need to be trained with lighter weight loads, medium to high repetitions, and markedly submaximal tensions, though continuous and isotensive.

For this reason, the table indicating the statistical percentages of the various muscle fibers found within a muscle can provide excellent indications for a training program.

Table of the percentage of various fibers in some muscles.

Muscle	% STa*	% FTa*	% FTb*
Adductor brevis	45	15	40
Brachial biceps	50	–	50
Femoral biceps	65	10	25
Deltoid	60	–	40
Gastrocnemius	50	20	30
Gracilis	55	15	30
Adductor magnus	55	15	30
Latissimus dorsi	50	–	50
Gluteus maximus	50	20	30
Pectoralis major	42	–	58
Iliopsoas	50	–	50
Psoas	50	20	30
Rectus abdominis	46	–	54
Rectus femoris	45	15	40
Rhomboid	45	–	55
Semimembranosus	50	15	35
Soleus	75	15	10
Tensor fascia lata	70	10	20
Tibialis anterior	70	10	20
Trapezius	54	–	64
Brachial triceps	33	–	67
Vastus intermedius	50	15	35
Vastus lateralis	45	20	35
Vastus medialis	50	15	35

* STa = Slow-twitch fibres
  FTA = Fast-twitch fibres
  FTB = Fast-twitch fibres

3.4 TYPES OF MUSCULAR CONTRACTION

Muscular contraction is defined as the physiological means through which muscular fibers are recruited once the nerve impulse has arrived and given a sufficient amount of energy. Muscular contractions divide into two groups: static contractions and dynamic contractions. In static contractions the muscle doesn't modify its length, even though tension is developed. Dynamic contractions determine, on the other hand, a modification in the muscle's length.

1. **Static (isometric) contractions.** The muscle develops an amount of tension equal to the resistance applied, doesn't modify its length (the distance between muscular insertions is unchanged), and doesn't generate any output (in the physical sense, meaning there is no displacement). Isometric contractions may be
   - maximal: tension is applied with an unmovable load; or
   - stationary: the movement is voluntarily interrupted.

2. **Dynamic (non-isometric) contractions.** The muscle develops tension and changes its length, producing an output; the distance between the insertions changes during contraction. Non-isometric contractions may be:
   - concentric (positive): the tension developed is such as to overcome the applied tension; the muscle shortens, and the insertions draw closer.
   - eccentric (negative): the tension developed is less than the resistance applied; the muscle lengthens, the insertions draw farther.
   - Isotonic: the muscle shortens, developing a constant tension for the entire length of the shortening period. Actually, in reality, isotonic contractions do not exist. The tension developed varies as the lever varies. We can simulate isotonic contraction only with machines featuring physiological camshafts.
   - Isokinetic: the muscle generates the maximum amount of tension throughout the movement, shortening at constant speed (specific isokinetic equipment is used).
   - Auxotonic: the tension generated increases progressively as the muscle shortens (e.g., an elastic band).
   - Plyometric: explosive, concentric contractions immediately preceded by eccentric contractions; this exploits the energy accumulated within the muscle's elastic structures.

CHAPTER

4

TRAINING THEORY

4.1   ORGANIC SYSTEMS

Our body has 11 systems. Each system is made up of different organs. These 11 systems are responsible for complex physical functions. In other words, each system has a specific goal. The physical functions are:

PROTECTION

1.   *Integumentary system:* the skin protects the underlying tissues, regulates body temperature, and synthesizes chemical substances and hormones.

SUPPORT AND MOVEMENT

1.   *Skeletal system.*
2.   *Muscular system.*

COMMUNICATIONS, CONTROL, AND INTEGRATION

1.   *Nervous system:* it takes care of the generation, transmission, integration, and gathering of specialized nerve impulses.
2.   *Endocrine system:* hormones are the main regulators of our metabolism, growth, development, reproduction, and other activities.

TRANSPORT AND DEFENSE

1. *Cardiovascular system.*
2. *Lymphatic system.*

TRANSFORMATION, REGULATION, AND MAINTENANCE

1. *Respiratory system.*
2. *Digestive system.*
3. *Urinary system:* kidneys cleanse waste from the blood. Inside the kidneys, the waste is transformed in urine.

REPRODUCTION AND GROWTH

1. *Reproductive system:* it guarantees the genetic code's survival.

All these systems exist in a state of equilibrium called homeostasis. The body constantly strives for equilibrium, reacting with negative feedback mechanisms to any sudden change.

Every time there is a sudden rise or fall in any system's parameters, the body activates certain physiological responses in order to bring the parameters back to the preexisting state of equilibrium.

Now, to avoid adopting the superior attitude of "experts" who train a different muscle group every day, you must understand that the stress applied on any system is also reflected on others and forces them to adapt.

Try this: Do a set of squats until you are exhausted. The effects? Respiration is fatigued, so therefore the cardiovascular and cardiorespiratory systems are stressed. The hip extensor chain—gluteus and quadriceps—is fatigued, and this means that the musculoskeletal system has been activated. Thighs and legs feel heavy, indicating the production of, the sign of an increased hormonal response (involving the endocrine system). We know also that among the physiological responses our body activates as a reaction to a stressful stimulus, such as training, there is an immune response. So another system is activated. Do you need to know more?

4.2   TRAINING: PRESENTATION

How to define training?

A person decides to start running, jumping, and doing push-ups with the arms and legs, doing this regularly until the onset of fatigue, trying to improve.

This means that this person is adding an extra energy stress (basal metabolism) to the daily energy consumption. This is not enough. This stress doesn't simply translate into greater energy consumption; it also translates into peripheral stress applied to the locomotor apparatus, which alters the equilibrium of the 11 organic systems that regulate this person's body. Sports training in physiology is defined as a stressor (i.e., a stressful stimulus). Compared to normal daily activities, stress is a series of factors that alter organic homeostasis, inducing a systemic response from the body. The systemic response is specific, depending on the type of stress involved, and non-specific, which is typical of all stress situations.

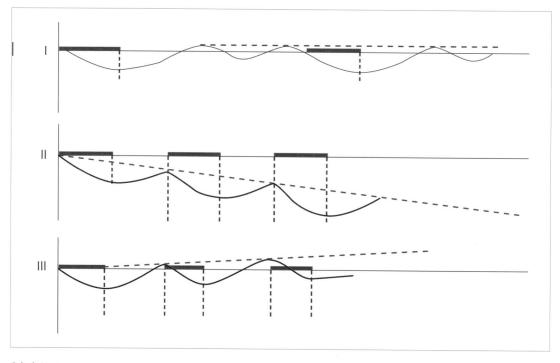

Selye's Law.

In order to be productive, stress must specifically have continuity (frequency), effort (intensity), and duration (volume). Training frequency determines the essential aspect that generates supercompensatory adaptations: recovery. This is what Selye's Law, or the law of supercompensation, says:

Following a stress situation, the organism activates a series of non-specific and specific responses involving the whole body, leading to a series of consequential adaptations after a suitable recovery.

The body effectively reacts to any stressful stimulus with a response and adaptation that are consequential and proportional to the stimulus received. Supercompensation will take place only after the organism has restored the conditions from before the onset of the training stress.

Improving a specific feature does not take place during the training session but during the following recovery phase; continuously subjecting someone to new training stress without allowing the body full recovery between sessions will cause overtraining syndrome (OTS).

4.3   TRAINING PROGRAM

Let's assume that training is the administration of stress, an additional burden to normal relational life that alters organic homeostasis in order to obtain a consequential response and adaptation (supercompensation).

In figure I (see page 58), the training stimulus is excessively rarefied.

This situation doesn't generate a chronic additional burden for the body, so there is no supercompensating adaptation.

In figure II, training stimuli which are excessively close to one another prevent supercompensating adaptation, quickly leading to overtraining.

In figure III, correctly scheduling training sessions over time leads to improvement.

You will notice in the definition of training the word *administration* is a pharmaceutical or medical term.

It was not chosen randomly. If training is to be scientific, its elaboration and training stimulus must be equally scientific.

Do remember: Each muscular structure has its own specific stimulus. This is a fact, even though it is true that certain stimuli, training for strength and its components, lead to improvement also in other structures, features, and characteristics.

Why? Any response is systemic: It involves the whole body.

Therefore a training program is the schedule of the stress (load) an individual must apply to his or her organic systems in order to obtain physiological modifications and related adaptations.

4.4 TRAINING THEORY

Let's now see which rules must be followed in order for training to yield results over time.

OVERLOAD

In order to induce physiological modifications leading to performance improvement, we must apply a training stimulus that is at least higher than that generated by normal daily life. This implies that once certain adaptations have been obtained, it will be necessary to train with workloads increasing in magnitude (load progressiveness) in order to further improve.

SPECIFICITY

A training stimulus will generate specific modifications in relation to the type of overload applied. Effectively, the benefits obtained from power training and those derived from aerobic training aren't interchangeable. In power training, we will have modifications typical of power training, while in aerobic training, there will be aerobic modifications.

INDIVIDUALITY

Given the multiple, infinite factors which differentiate one person from another, it isn't advisable to apply the same training program to all people, using identical stimuli, loads, and exercises. Training must be programmed according to the person , bearing in mind his or her physical, structural, and metabolic characteristics.

LOSS OF TRAINING

The effects of training are transitory and reversible proportional to the type, intensity, and duration of the applied stimulus. After 10-14 days of rest, there is a regression in several motor components already achieved.

4.5   TRAINING PARAMETERS

PLANNING

Plan training type and load rationally according to the amounts required by a specific discipline and by the goals to be reached in a well-defined time period. This takes place by structuring physical exercise in amounts and intensities that will provide progressively increasing workloads in order to stimulate the physiological processes of adaptation and supercompensation.

VOLUME

Volume represents the amount of work carried out during a workout unit. It is measured in different ways, according to the discipline referred to.

In bodybuilding, the total work volume is usually identified by the number of sets executed or the training session duration and by each muscle group's specific work volume (repetitions) or the time spent stimulating that same muscle.

INTENSITY

This is perhaps the most debated parameter and an object of disagreement between different schools of thought.

Definitions and formulas which are valid for performance sports aren't well suited to an anomalous discipline such as bodybuilding. In weight training, training intensity is directly related to the amount of kg [lb] lifted:

$$I = Kg\ [lb] \times R/\ T$$

I = Intensity
Kg [lb]= Kg [lb] lifted
R = Repetitions performed
T = Time needed to complete the set

This formula expresses a measure of power, since:

$$Kg\ [lb] \times R$$

merely represents Work.

The work carried out in the Time unit expresses Power, but intensity isn't simply identifiable as the measure of the power output.

Intensity is the type of effort with which a certain gesture is carried out, implying a strong subjective component which is hard to measure.

- According to Prof. Emilio They, training intensity depends on the amount of motor units involved in the unit of time between a 0-degree and a 180-degree angle (extension) or between a 180-degree and a 0-degree angle (flexion).
- Intensity is a value related to the neurophysiologic mechanism of recruitment of the various motor units, and it is not necessarily related to weight, repetitions, and duration. It is therefore a personal and contingent factor which is not measurable through external data.

Intensity in a bodybuilding exercise is given by:

$$I = IC/N \times 100$$

I = Intensity
IC = Intensity coefficient
N = Total number of repetitions performed

While executing a set, you count the number of repetitions performed from the time when real fatigue sets in. This number is the Intensity coefficient (IC). When all is taken into account, the intensity parameter is probably the most important factor in training. There is a level of intensity below which there are no biological modifications inside the muscle; it is only a waste of time.

4.6   EXERCISES

Exercises are the means of training. They are the movements through which stress is administered by applying loads to the organic levers.

Choosing the correct exercises implies evaluating their effectiveness.

Let's distinguish between complex exercises, or general conditioning exercises, and competition exercises, or specific exercises (which reproduce a specific athletic movement). In athletic training, complex exercises are used to strengthen the whole locomotor apparatus, the conditioning abilities, and motor qualities.

Competition exercises instead reproduce or imitate the technically athletic gesture typical of a sporting performance. In physical education, this concept is simplified, and we prefer to differentiate between basic exercises and complementary exercises.

4.6.1   Complex exercises

FEATURES AND FUNCTIONS

- They are multiarticular.
- They work on long kinematic chains.
- They have great muscular synergy.
- They have a straight trajectory.
- There is greater external load (lifted weight).
- There is greater internal load (the external load's effects on the body).
- There is greater recruitment of motor units.
- It has great systemic response (endocrine, lymphatic, circulatory, immune).
- It is essential for ectomorphic subjects.
- It has great hormonal response.

RECOMMENDED USE

- In the initial stages of fitness training (the fundamentals).
- In the general conditioning phase, where they must make up at least 70% of the training elements.
- As strength mesocycles.
- As hypertrophy mesocycles.
- During the pre-competition phase, where they must make up at least 30% of the training elements.
- In slimming programs.

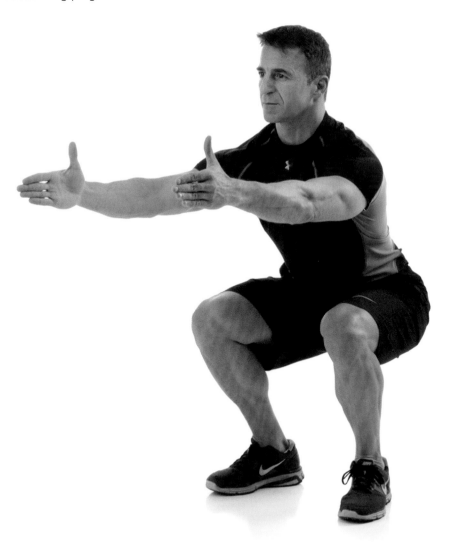

4.6.2   Competition exercises

FEATURES AND FUNCTIONS

- They are monoarticular.
- They generate a pinpointed, localized, targeted stimulus.
- They have low muscular synergy.
- There is a curved trajectory.
- There is greater muscular stretching (protein synthesis increases, both *in vivo* and *in vitro*).
- There is a lower hormonal response (a slight increase in GH).
- It has qualitative movement (i.e., correct, technical movements).
- It has low synergy.

RECOMMENDED USE

- In pre-competition phase.
- As hypertrophy mesocycles.
- In overload, high-intensity techniques.
- In highly sedentary, obese, or strongly overweight subjects.
- When working on specific areas.
- In postural training.
- In physical therapy training.

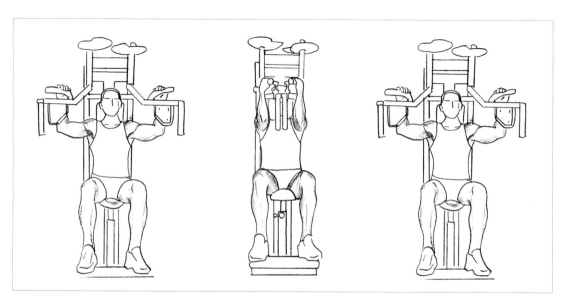

Given the high organic response they create, only basic exercises truly determine the greater effectiveness of a training program. Their prevailing factor is quantitative (i.e., the load). Complementary exercises have a mainly qualitative character, especially in the course of the specific training phase. In gyms, we must distinguish between, if you will, major league and minor league complementary exercises. Let me explain: In the weights room, we don't have a technical performance objective, and it is therefore important to concentrate on those complementary exercises which yield greater muscle stretching. Stretching, both in vivo and in vitro, can in fact increase protein synthesis and induce interesting adaptations.

FUNCTIONAL TRAINING

5.1   KINETIC AND KINEMATIC CHAINS

In human articular physiology, monoarticular movements do not exist. We could perform them, but they aren't the priority for the locomotor apparatus. For economy and practicality, our body uses complex movements almost exclusively. In physics, *kinetic chain* is a system of rigid segments connected by mobile joints called junctions.

Our body is made up of many kinetic chains that are set off by our muscles. With the term *katakinetics* (Payr[1], 1936) or *kinematic chain* (Reuleux[2], 1934), we refer to the set of organs and systems that determine the human body's voluntary movements.

- By open *kinetic chain* we mean a system in which the furthermost end (the distal end) is free and unconstrained. Example: the lower limbs when walking.
- A closed *kinetic chain* is when the distal end is fixed. In other words, it cannot move during the execution of the gesture without involving another chain. Examples: squats or horizontal bench exercises.

---

1 Hanfried K. (2004). On the Development of the Constraint Motion Theory of Franz Reuleaux – An Overview, in *International Symposium on History of Machines and Mechanisms*, pp. 201-215.

2 Hanfried K. (2004). On the Development of the Constraint Motion Theory of Franz Reuleaux – An Overview, in *International Symposium on History of Machines and Mechanisms*, pp. 201-215.

5.2   THE MEANING OF FUNCTIONAL

The term *functional* is very trendy nowadays, with meanings ranging from A to Z. It's like an empty tube anyone can fill up as he or she pleases with everything and nothing. Our objective is to start with a scientific definition, without which it would be impossible to build a methodology.

Let's clear any misunderstandings by working with the dictionary definition.

From the Oxford English Dictionary, Functional: of or serving a function; designed or intended to; having a function.

You can't get any clearer...

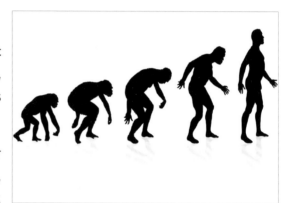

Functional training is a form of training that is related to the function for which a muscle, or rather a kinematic chain, exists and has evolved in a certain way.

The evolutionary choices of our locomotor apparatus explain the function of each muscle, kinematic chain, and articular system in our body.

How do we apply this concept?

a)   by adapting it to each subject's articular structure.
b)   by adapting it to the functions of the muscles or the kinematic chains which are activated.

The definition of functional training as training related to the function of the muscles in the course of a normal daily life isn't correct.

A reference parameter is actually missing: whose daily life? A weightlifting athlete's? A white-collar worker's? A sedentary person's? Daily life is different from person to person, but each one of us has the same kinematic chains.

5.3   THE ACTION-FUNCTION PRINCIPLE

The evolution in modern training is to train each muscle according to its action (a principle which is frequently applied in gyms) and to its function (a feature which is often neglected).

We must start by understanding the evolutionary choices of our locomotor apparatus.

Gyms have emphasized the concept of isolation to the extreme, focusing attention purely on muscular action but losing sight of the whole—the reason why that specific muscle, kinetic, or articular chain has evolved in a certain way.

From this stems the action-function principle:

The training of each motor feature or skill must be programmed on the basis of the action and function of the kinematic chain to which it is applied.

Without this type of programming, any training will inevitably be incomplete.

To simplify:

Functional training = Action + Function

For the same reason, functional exercises can hardly be defined as pectoralis, latissimus dorsi, or quadriceps exercises.

By working on kinematic chains as extensively as possible, large muscular areas will be engaged, even though one specific section will benefit the most.

The objective of functional training is systemic stress, involving as many organic systems as possible. This isn't enough. Understanding the evolutional changes which made us as we are today will help us understand how and why a specific muscle has developed a certain function and, consequently, how best to train it.

5.4 PEBBLES INTO A POND

Only by engaging the concept of functional training can we appreciate the shocking errors made in the development of exercises and methodologies which concentrate (often mistakenly) only on one aspect of training: action.

A few examples:

1. The femoral biceps and hamstring group
There are four muscular bands:

- Short end of the femoral biceps.
- Long end of the femoral biceps.
- Semimembranosus.
- Semitendinosus.

Of the four, only one is monoarticular: the short end of the femoral biceps. The action is flexing the lower leg to the thigh. The three others are biarticular, as they ride across the knee and hip joints. The actions are flexing the leg to the thigh and extending the thigh from the pelvis.

As stated in chapter 1, biarticular muscles must be stimulated with biarticular movements to be fully trained. In a gym there are no biarticular machines for the femoral biceps. Following the principles of biomechanics, training on the iconic leg curl machines, the only machines specific for this group, will always be incomplete.

Let's look into the function of the femoral group to discover which exercises will train it. For more information, refer to chapter 6 on the hip extensor chain.

2. The adductor group
The adductor group has three monoarticular bands and one biarticular one: the gracilis. The adductor's action is to adduct the lower limbs. The gracilis muscle adducts the thigh and flexes and medially turns the leg. The sartorius originates in the anterior part of the thigh; it is thus a part of the adductor group, but it acts synergistically with the gracilis (and with the femoral group, since it flexes the thigh to the pelvis), as flexor of the leg on the thigh.

In a gym these muscles are trained, especially in women, on the classic adductor machines. Let's think about it: Do we have our evolutionary choices in mind? Monkeys, from which we derive, all have the adductor group, yet we have never seen a monkey open and close its legs in any instance in daily life. It's evident that we have lost sight of this muscle group's function, and its training is therefore incomplete. What is the adductor group's function? The adductor is a muscle with the function of acting as a stabilizer; it's also a flexor and an extensor, according to the position of its contralateral limb. It must therefore be trained with multijoint movements, using body weight.

3. Abdominal fascia: The core

This is probably the worst-trained area in the history of weight training. In gyms, core training has become a saga: a thousand and one ways of doing crunches! As with the previous point: monkeys have the abdominal fascia, as we do, but do not perform crunch movements. It's clear, then, that the abdominal fascia has other functions besides the one we train with simple abdominal floor exercises. We must not forget we are bipeds and that our customary position is, or at least ought to be, standing. If we think about it, it is intuitive that the main function of the abdominal fascia cannot be that which is performed by exercising supine on the ground. We are now ready to answer these and other questions about functional training.

5.5   OBJECTIVES

The purpose of functional training is to totally develop conditional and motor skills and motor. In simple terms, we try to train an athlete who has a propensity for strength and endurance. In other words, this athlete displays hypertrophy that isn't purely aesthetic and disappears at the first cold, but it is functional. It is useful', so our locomotor apparatus will not easily do without it.

In addition, be defined as a strength and endurance athlete, an individual must have certain body composition parameters (unless the specific performance activity directs him or her toward different weight choices). Our athlete must therefore pay attention to nutrition and supplementation. He or she must also develop various coordination abilities, beginning with proprioception (perhaps the most important one), in order to prevent injuries and optimize performance.

5.5.1   What are the benefits of functional training?

Functional training is:

More adapted to organic physiology

a)   it emphasizes the relationship between the locomotor apparatus and the environment.

b)   in younger subjects and particularly in older ones, it optimizes the synthesis of vitamin D (the lack of which leads to an increased risk of fractures).

c)   it allows all 11 endogenous systems to activate spontaneously.

d)   it takes place mostly in the standing position. How often do we forget we are bipeds? And yet, statistically, we stand for only two hours a day. Presumably the bodyweight load at the lumbar level is the main cause of back aches.

More functional

a)   because you do it standing up (an athlete always ought to train standing!).

b)   because it activates long kinematic chains.

c)   because it trains muscular chains according to the action-function combination.

d)   because it trains all of the coordination skills.

e)   because it follows our evolutionary history.

More effective for training compared to the classic indoor disciplines

a)   in biomechanical terms.

b)   in muscular terms.

c)   in terms of the endogenous systems involved.

Let's just think about the difference between running on a treadmill and running on a road or dirt track.

In terms of muscular engagement, when running on a treadmill we do have the eccentric phase of the movement but the concentric phase—the extension of the thigh on the pelvis—is performed by the treadmill's own rotation, partially blocking the full motion of the gluteus. Furthermore, the foot strike is cushioned by the machine. The simple impact of the foot on the ground (not necessarily bumpy or unpaved) during a run or a walk outdoors has magnified consequences from a biomechanical point of view, and it also trains proprioception.

Also consider the work done using a road bike or a mountain bike compared to that done in a gym on vertical or horizontal stationary bikes.

5.6 MOTIVATIONS

The objective of functional training is to create athletes, forming our bodies into personalized outfits.

Another outcome of functional training makes it unique. Our motivation to become more fit on the outside goes hand in hand with improvements at the physical level. The more a person appreciates the progress and the strengthening of the organic systems (cardiorespiratory, endocrine, lymphatic, musculotendinous), the more that person will become mentally stronger, more determined, motivated and efficient. He or she will train in increasingly demanding conditions (rain, cold weather), with increasingly more intense activities (uphill and downhill running exercises, forest exercises).

Whoever said that functional, body-weight exercises are easy? Challenge yourselves on dirt tracks, beaches, meadows, or any other outdoor or indoor surface. Execute walking lunges for only 100 m (109.4 yd) because it doesn't matter how long you take; you can stop, rest, catch your breath...and then carry on!

Three days or a week later, return to the "scene of crime" and do the same exercise, but try one of three things differently:

1. Cover the same distance in a shorter time.
2. Take the same time but increase the distance covered.
3. Take less time and increase the distance.

Trying is believing!

5.7 FUNCTIONAL TRAINING AND PRE-ATHLETICISM

The term *pre-athleticism* can have two meanings:

1. Development of the athletic components in a child during the growth phase.
2. Training for specific performance sports.

And even a third new meaning, the one we refer to, about generic pre-athleticism or general physical preparation (GPP):

3. Multilateral work structured for the development of motor and coordinative abilities functional to a general psycho–physical enhancement.

In terms of this, Hirtz's[3] (1985) model identifies seven coordinative abilities:

1. Kinesthetic differentiation ability.
2. Movement combination and segmental coordination ability.
3. Reaction ability.
4. Orientation ability.
5. Balancing ability.
6. Adaptation and transformation ability.
7. Rhythmic ability.

To these general abilities we can add three others:

8. Motor learning ability.
9. Movement control ability.
10. Movement variation ability.

GPP work is, for the majority of athletes, the secret for working functionally and for wearing one's body like a dress.

Functional training will allow you to climb the steps of physical efficiency, while at the same time developing all those qualities which constitute the basis for it.

---

3 Hirtz P. (1985). *Coordination Abilities in School Sports*. Volk und Wissen.

5.8 FUNCTIONAL TRAINING: OTHER FACTORS TO DEVELOP

5.8.1 Training recruitment

Training recruitment means working on the central nervous system. The best age to obtain established improvements in this sense is before 14; specific training beyond this age will, however, improve several factors in recruitment, both spatial and temporal, though with a semi-automatic acquisition.

EXAMPLE 1

A child learns to ski and then, for whatever reason, doesn't practice this activity for a few years. When the child puts the skis back on, he or she will ski as well as before stopping (it will only be necessary to reacquire confidence).

EXAMPLE 2

An adult learns to ski with perseverance and frequency then, for whatever reason, doesn't practice for years. When the adult puts the skis back on, he or she will have to start almost from the beginning again (the stoppage time factor is significant).

Let's distinguish between spatial and temporal recruitment:

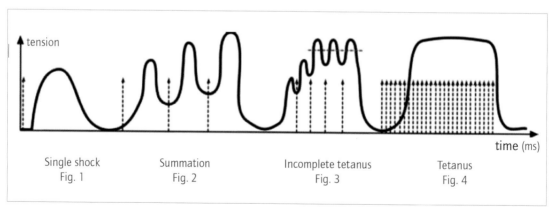

Summation

- **Spatial recruitment:** it is the increase in the number of motor units recruited during contraction and can be one of two types:

1. *progressive:* strength is developed gradually along the time scale (imagine pressing the foot down gradually on a car accelerator).
2. *ballistic:* the command signal reaches the muscle in a tiny window of approximately 100 ms (Paillard, 1982). Imagine flooring the accelerator immediately and hard.

- **Temporal recruitment:** it's the increase in the discharge frequency by the nervous system (via summation).

  - When a motor signal is sent by the central nervous system to a single fiber, the fiber first contracts then releases (fig. 1).
  - When the motor message is transmitted more effectively by increasing the impulse frequency, the tension generated by the muscle increases through the summation effect of two closely-spaced impulses (fig. 2).
  - With several closely-spaced impulses, the tension produced will increase further as a result of their summation, the clonus condition (fig. 3).
  - Beyond this limit, if the impulse frequency increases still, the maximum possible tension, called the tetanus, is developed (fig. 4).

5.8.1.1   Training recruitment in adults

It is possible to train the central nervous system, hence training recruitment, in adults. The objective is to increase neuromuscular activation by performing exercises outside the usual criteria:

- **More complex exercises:** involving long chains and working with several body districts together in order to force the central nervous system to engage in a higher effort.
- *Uncomfortable, destabilizing exercises:* using unconventional or differentiated equipment, making the execution more difficult; working from a standing position with differentiated loads, involving the body's stabilizing systems and muscles.

- **Plyometric and isometric contractions:** alternate to the normal concentric and eccentric phases. Varying the type of contraction within the same exercise has an uncommon training impact.
- **Working on the muscle's elastic components:** with exercises which involve a pre-stretching of the muscle trained (i.e., pulling away its origin and insertion). We forget that working with these factors is inside us—it is part of primitive activities such as running, walking, jumping, and sprinting.
- **Functional exercises:** training the muscles according to the action-function principle.

5.8.2   Strengthening pivot muscles

Whatever its objectives, training must reinforce pivot muscles for preventative and also performance improvement purposes. By pivot we mean those muscle groups belonging mainly to the deep musculature with the main function of joint stabilization—muscles which are loaded with tension during exercise performance.

The main ones are:

- Rotator cuff
- Flexors and extensors of the forearm and fingers
- Periscapular muscles
- Wide abdominal muscles
- Paravertebral muscles
- Tibial and adductor muscles
- Triceps surae muscle

When building an athlete, training these groups must take precedence over training others.

5.8.3   Reinforcing the weak links in the kinematic chains

It is of utmost importance when training to remember in a kinematic chain, the weakest muscle influences the functionality of the entire chain. If we have a chain made of several iron links and one paper link, the paper link will be the first to give way, and because of its frailty, will weaken the whole chain. Working on kinematic chains allows us to examine the weakest muscular links and to work on strengthening them using

- chains,
- elastics bands,
- kettlebells,
- sandbags,
- medicine balls, and
- shortened movements with supports.

Contrary to common wisdom, work on the weak link should not be aimed at hypertrophy. We must always take into account the synergy of the muscles involved in the same chain.

5.8.4   Breaking the pattern

This is one of the most interesting aspects of functional training: the ability to progress in a thousand different directions, to apply a variety of stimuli which gym activity cannot provide. Any structure, any object, whether natural or not—a tree, a branch, a rock, a rising slope, a flight of steps, a sand or cement sack, a wood, a beach, a track, a meadow, a dirt track, a low wall—can become the center of new workouts, new exercises, or new applications of the same.

The first step in breaking the pattern and building a motor map as wide as possible is to stimulate the central nervous system with basic exercise programs and unconventional exercises—the key principle being movement variation. And change an exercise not session by session but set by set, within the same session.

Every time we subject our central nervous system (and consequently the locomotor apparatus) to a new type of movement, we apply stress to it. At this stage, the central nervous system will be forced to adapt and enhance all the systems involved, owing to the continuity and repetition of the movement. A body which is prodded by multiple stimuli will be always proactive, ready to change; it will be able to react and adapt much more quickly. Variability of movement is the central nervous system's oil (Guido Veestagen[4], 2014).

As an example of what we mean, let's describe an exercise and its progression set by set:

1. Walking lunge.
2. Asymmetric walking lunge (weight on one arm only).
3. Walking lunge with two dumbbells.
4. Overhead walking lunge (one arm lifts the weight above the head).

Working on long kinematic chains, for example, is almost unknown in gyms, excepting squats and deadlifts. These are typical weightlifting technical gestures in which, after the loading phase, the weight is heaved upward and the body is simultaneously lowered in the opposite direction, fitting underneath the load. They are extremely difficult for the average gym patron, who is used to heavy loads but extremely simple exercises.

---

4 Veestagen G., (2010-2012-2014). Personal communication, *Perform Better Convention*, LA.

CHAPTER 6

HIP EXTENSOR CHAIN

6.1 PRESENTATION

Ask any athletics coach from Eastern European countries or the US: "Where does the secret of strength lie? Where does it come from?" They will reply: "From the hips, from the hip extensor chain". Hip muscles express strength and power more so than other muscles. It is not a coincidence part of the hip extensor chain is the gluteus, the human body's strongest muscle (after the masseter, the chewing muscle). Think of any performance sport and you will see that in some way this chain is deeply involved in it.

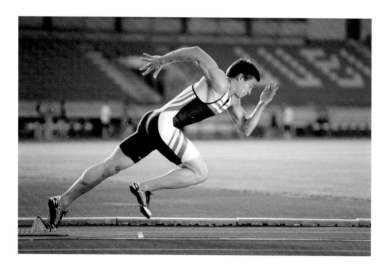

Training the lower limbs has a great importance in terms of prevention and pre-athleticism, even more than aesthetics. Studies provide ample confirmation of this when training is supported by basic exercises. Let's start with what we know: Ample articular excursions in the lower limbs (i.e., full squats) determine significant hormonal distress (Bosco[1] and coll., 1996).

It is clear then: the lower limb training bastions (squats, leg presses, sagittal lunges, deadlifts) do work. Their combined use satisfies any and all needs for strength, tone, and muscular tropism. But the question we must ask ourselves is: do they train thighs and glutes completely? The answer is no! These exercises actually train the gluteus, the quadriceps, and in general the lower limb muscles according to their action and the flexion and extension of the thigh on the pelvis, but not their function.

Do we remember the concept of functional training? It is Action + Function. What is the function of the gluteus? It is propulsion.

Now take a look around gyms, and you will notice that there are no exercises featuring propulsion or that work with propulsion in any way.

In the training this chain, exercises in which this thrusting action is present are missing, such as

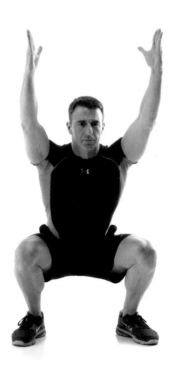

- jumps,
- skips,.
- plyometric jumps,
- uphill walking,
- sprinting (better if uphill),
- starter exercises,
- swing exercises, and
- ballistic exercises.

Functional training = Action + Function

Let's never forget it.

---

1 Bosco C. and Viru A. (1996) *Biologia dell'allenamento*, SSS, Roma

6.2 ACTION AND FUNCTION OF THE LOWER BODY

The function of the coxofemoral joint and of the muscles which originate or are inserted nearby confirm the necessity for functional training of the lower body.

The muscles in the joints of the lower body contrast the effect of gravity and of any other force that tends to destabilize the body's balance.

The functions of the lower-body muscles are:

- Double support in the upright stance.
- Oscillation and support during locomotion.
- Transfer of the body from a lying down to an upright position.
- Sensitive information from the support points.

During ambulation, when one leg is lifted, the hip muscles are active in shifting the body weight onto the support limb and preventing the pelvis from falling down the side which isn't supported.

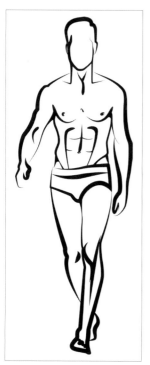

ADDUCTORS

They contract to shift the pelvis toward the support side; furthermore, they can act as hip extensors or flexors when walking or running, according to whether they are forward or behind the rotation axis. Finally, they stabilize the pelvis.

ABDUCTORS

When walking and running, they stabilize the pelvis on the support side, preventing it from falling.

ILIOPSOAS

It rotates the pelvis forward and is active in walking, climbing stairs, running or walking uphill, and getting up from a supine position.

QUADRICEPS

When running, it helps the gluteus to realize its maximal potential in the final extension phase.

GLUTEUS MAXIMUS

It is the body's most powerful muscle, the largest (66 cm2 [25.9 in2] in section) and the strongest. Its main action is the extension of the thigh on the pelvis. Its function is propulsion. This muscle is indispensable when running, jumping, and marching uphill.

FEMORAL BICEPS, SEMITENDINOSUS, AND SEMIMEMBRANOSUS

The femoral muscle group had already been reevaluated by the athletic training schools in Eastern European countries, and these evaluations are shared by American athletics coaches. It is a group of biarticular muscles (except for the short end of the femoral biceps), that ride the knee joint distally and the coxofemoral joint proximately. As such, their main action is the extension of the thigh on the pelvis, in synergy with the gluteus maximus, to which they also offer a great functional support in propulsion.

PIRIFORMIS MUSCLE

It is a hip abductor. Its action is maximized at a 60-degree flexion of the hip. It has an external rotation action before reaching 60degrees of flexion and an internal rotation one beyond 60 degrees. Pivoting on the femur, the piriformis inclines the pelvis contralaterally and tilts it backward. The piriformis is important because of its close contact with the sciatic nerve. Symptoms such as sciatic pains similar to those found in cases of herniated discs are frequent and attributed to an excessive shortening of this small muscle; curiously, they are also called "wallet-in-the-back-pocket syndrome", since the habit of wearing such objects seems to lead to articular compression and the shortening of the piriformis.

From this we can deduce that the main action of the coxofemoral joint and therefore of the whole hip extensor chain is propulsion. In order for the training of this kinematic chain to be complete, then, following the action-function principle, we have to add to basic and multijoint exercises of proven effectiveness (e.g., squats and lunges) and other exercises in which this function is expressed.

6.3 ARTICULAR REALITY: LONG-LIMBED AND SHORT-LIMBED SUBJECTS

We said at the beginning that articular reality, which varies from individual to individual, is an expression of functionality and therefore of evolutionary choices.

Among articular systems, the coxofemoral is the one that most exemplifies this evolution. Anthropologists have in fact noted how the shape of the femur—diaphysis, neck, and head—responds exactly to these evolutionary criteria. Its shape is variable and depends on functional adjustments. We can therefore distinguish two different types: the long-limbed subject and the short-limbed subject (Bellugue, P., 1963).

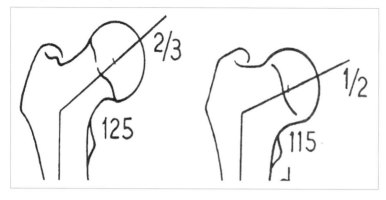

Femur head in long-limbed and short-limbed subjects (picture from Kapandji).

LONG-LIMBED TYPE

The femur head is a sphere 4-5 cm [1.5-1.8 in] in diameter for more than two thirds of the femur, supported by the femur neck which binds it to the diaphysis.

The femur neck axis forms with its diaphysial axis a tilt angle of 125 degrees and a declination angle of 25 degrees with the frontal plane.

The femoral diaphysis is thin, and the pelvis is small and high. This combination means a wide articular excursion of the femur head within the articular cavity, and this ensures great articular width, which can mean a talent for running. This subject is therefore suited to this type of activity (think of the Kenyan marathon runners).

SHORT-LIMBED TYPE

The femur head is barely larger than a half of a sphere; the tilt angle of the femur neck corresponds to 115 degrees, while the declination angle is about 10 degrees. The femoral diaphysis is short and thick. This combination means a limited amount of femur head excursion within its articular cavity. It is a morphology of strength. What the subject loses in terms of speed, he or she regains in strength and power.

6.3.1   Consequences

A specific anthropometric trait corresponds to a characteristic biotype.

Without dwelling too much on this, when we talk about biotype (from the Greek *bios* and *tupos*, meaning life print), we mean a group of individuals with similar physical, hormonal, personality, and other features. **The long-limbed type,** also called ectomorphs, is only slightly hypertrophic in both upper and lower body. It is an adrenaline-sensitive subject, with high levels of catecholamines and thyroid hormones and low levels of testosterone and androgens. It is poorly suited for weight training and tires easily and quickly.

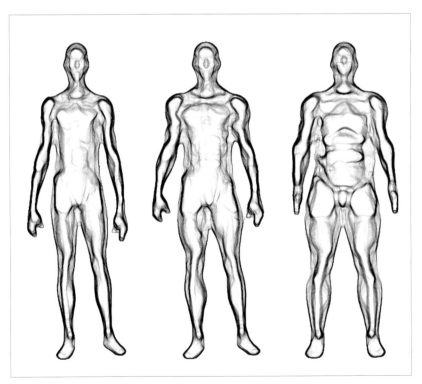

Ectomorphic, mesomorphic, endomorphic.

Training for this subject will need to be exclusively focused on long kinematic chains, involving large muscular areas; the training ought to incorporate the classic basic exercises and functional movements that are expressions of strength and power (skips, vertical and plyometric jumps, one-legged jumps). This is because we need to induce a strong hormonal response, especially at the androgen level, through training.

The short-limbed type, endomorph, has a greater propensity to upper- and lower-body hypertrophy. Generally, it has a low metabolism, great muscular mass and strength but also a propensity to gain weight. The female subject will have to pace herself in the basic exercises and include functional movements with aspects of endurance (uphill walking or walking) that do not involve white fibers. The male subject will easily increase muscular mass and will have to concentrate on slimming. A typical training program could feature one day of total body weights, one or two of circuit training, and possibly one day exclusively dedicated to aerobic work.

6.4 BACK ACHE, THE ILIOPSOAS, AND EVOLUTION

Evolutionary choices form the basis of functional training and explain the adaptations and changes our body has gone throughin the course of millennia. What we are today is the result of those choices. What is amusing is that we never think of ourselves as an outcome. So to speak, 6.5 million years ago we were a bunch of Australopithecines. The achievement of the upright posture is supposed to date back to about 2.5 million years ago. It represented a huge leap along the evolutionary scale. To explain this better: The life of an anthropomorphic monkey takes place over 10 square miles, while our hominid ancestor could cover this distance in just one day when hunting for food. Then followed the reversal of mandibular prognathism.

Coming to the present age, it is clear that evolutionary choices have always had biological and physiological justifications (we are, after all, the dominant species on the planet). We must proceed from here and think about the current issues. The most common pathologies in bone and joint muscular terms are back pains, especially at the sacral-lumbar level. The vertebrae that are statistically most affected are L5-S1 and L4-L5. At the heart of these aches there is almost always an excessive retraction of the hip flexors. The shortening of the iliopsoas—and even more common in sporting subjects, of the rectus femoris—is responsible for a more or less pronounced hyperlordosis; this attitude is favored by hypotonia of the rectus abdominis. The number one cause of these retractions is a sedentary life. Look at small children, and you will notice that they execute perfect squats with complete ease, and they easily hold a full crouch. Similar adaptations are still to be found today in several people on various continents. We have forgotten that man has evolved as a biped and as such must functionally discharge tensions and loads to the ground through a system of joints and shock absorbers: the joint capsules. The problem is that today, so statistics say, we stand up for only two hours a day and for the rest of the time we sit down on chairs, stools, seats, and sofas. A sedentary lifestyle doesn't fit with the evolutionary processes, albeit only progressively in older subjects. In all of these non-physiological positions, the support point for the locomotor apparatus is the pelvis in the sacral area. This is where we discharge forces and tensions for eight, ten, and even more hours every day, causing neuromuscular retractions as well. We could then ask why our body has chosen to preserve the iliopsoas despite all the problems it causes. We know that it is an important muscle for walking and running, according to Delmas' spinal index, but this feature has become more pronounced after coming down from the trees.

What about before? Why was it already there before? What is the function of the iliopsoas? We can use the following example to find the answer. A young man in a gym is performing chin-ups. For the first few repetitions, it all goes well; the body is perpendicular to the ground, and the execution is correct. Then fatigue sets in. What does our subject do? He bends the thighs into the pelvis. Why? Because in doing so he shortens the lever's arm and manages to complete a few more repetitions. Monkeys, from which we descended, execute the same movement when they move from one branch to another: They stretch and extend in the aerial phase, and shorten themselves by flexing their thighs and trunk during the traction phase. Also, when chimpanzees walk, they lean forward with their trunks and diminish the lordosis of their lower backs. Remember that the psoas muscle creates lordosis in the back by arching it. Monkeys keep using the iliopsoas, but they start from a lengthening position. Probably humankind has not yet adapted to the upright posture, and this would explain the dichotomy between the psoas function on the one hand and the use we make of it on the other. In general, seeing the difference between their action-function and current use, I believe it is always best to train these muscles by stretching them.

CHAPTER 7

ABDOMINAL FASCIA

7.1 PRESENTATION

When we talk about the abdominal fascia, we are discussing the most important area for the health of the bone-joint apparatus. The relevance of this whole area has come increasingly more important so that you frequently hear about core training. The abdominal segment connects the trunk and the lower limbs. The lumbar-pelvic region consists of:

- 35 bilateral muscles inserted in the pelvis.
- 14 muscles that link the pelvis to the spine.
- 21 muscles that connect the pelvis to the lower extremities.

*The abdominal corset
(picture from Kapandji[1]).*

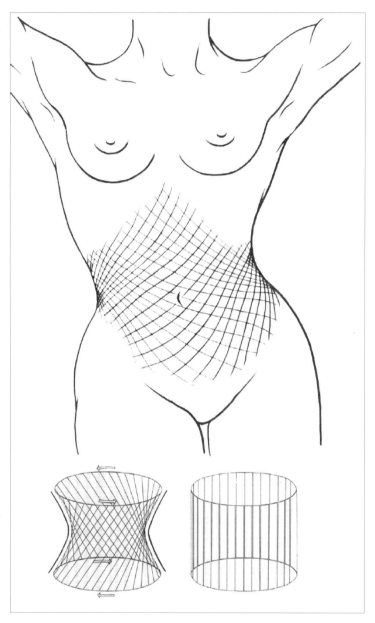

In the course of evolution, the rachis has changed from being a link between upper, anterior limbs and lower, posterior limbs to an antigravity support structure with static and dynamic features. In the presence of hypotonia of the rachis musculature, we assume incorrect and deficient postures which may lead to spine problems, such as postural defects, or pathologies, such as hyperlordosis, hyperkyfosis, or worse, scoliosis. A strong athlete will have a strong abdomen and toned, efficient abdominal fascia.

1 Kapandji I.A (1983). *The Physiology of the Joints*, Elsevier Churchill Livingstone Publisher.

89

7.2   CORE

The functions of the abdominal fascia are stabilization, motion, and control. But we are specifically talking about these muscles:

- Rectus abdominis
- Transversus abdominis.
- Internal oblique muscles.
- External oblique muscles.
- Quadratus lumborum.
- Erector spinae.
- Pelvic floor muscles.

We may think of the core as a bucket. The cylindrical supporting structure consists of three strata of muscles: the transversus abdominis and the oblique muscles. The anterior securing hinge is the rectus abdominis, and the posterior hinge is made of the erector spinae muscles and the quadratus lumborum. The bottom of the bucket is made by the pelvic floor muscles.

7.3   PELVIC FLOOR

The pelvic floor is a group of muscles which creates a weave among the pelvis bones. In the course of evolution, with the shift from a horizontal, quadrupedal or semi-quadrupedal posture to the upright posture, the pelvic floor muscles have decidedly changed their function. If before their almost exclusive function was waste expulsion and synergy in parturition, now with the bipedal posture they have acquired the role of support platform for the organs and the abdominal cavity. In the female subject, the poor activation of pelvic floor muscles is the cause of frequent pathologies, especially post-childbirth complications, from incontinence to the prolapse (a collapse) of the uterus.

7.4   ACTION OF THE ABDOMINAL FASCIA

The core's complexity relates primarily to its muscles.

RECTUS ABDOMINIS

This muscle flexes the trunk forward and laterally; it raises the pelvis and participates in abdominal pressure. It plays an important role in maintaining the correct posture of the pelvis, as an antagonist to the quadratus lumborum. It is a muscle with an important aesthetic value, but, functionally speaking, it is secondary to the large abdominal muscles.

EXTERNAL OBLIQUE MUSCLE

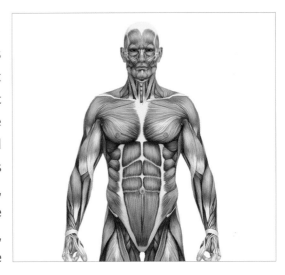

This muscle is synergistic to the rectus abdominis in the flexing of the trunk. It tilts the trunk laterally and turns it contralaterally (the right external oblique muscle turns the trunk to the left, and vice versa). It participates in the final rotation extension in all the throwing movements practiced in athletics such as rugby, tennis, baseball, golf, and even boxing. Every time we apply a weight to one side of the body (e.g., carrying a suitcase or a dumbbell), the oblique muscles on the opposite side contract in order to stabilize the trunk and prevent it from falling laterally. It is part of the abdominal corset.

INTERNAL OBLIQUE MUSCLE

This muscle shares in the forward flexion of the trunk; it tilts the trunk laterally or turns it toward the contracting side. In rotation, it is synergistic with the rectus abdominis and the external oblique muscle on the opposite side. It contributes to abdominal pressure.

TRANSVERSUS ABDOMINIS

This muscle's main activity is abdominal pressure: It holds back the viscera and stabilizes the pelvis. It is thanks to the synergy between the transversus abdominis and the oblique muscles that the pelvis and the lumbar tract acquire strength and stability.

QUADRATUS LUMBORUM

As the name itself suggests (*quadratus* means "square" in Latin), this is a square-shaped muscle that goes from the iliac crest to the spine and the ribs. It tilts the trunk backward and laterally. It is the real antagonist of the rectus abdominis.

ERECTOR SPINAE AND LATISSIMUS DORSI

Their action is the extension and lateral tilt of the back.

7.5 FUNCTION OF THE ABDOMINAL FASCIA

Let's start talking about the function of the abdominal fascia muscles beginning from the synergy between the diaphragmatic and the mediastinal cavities that border each other. They are physically divided but functionally associated. With inspiration, when the thorax expands, the mediastinal cavity is depressed; with expiration it is the diaphragmatic cavity which is depressed, while the mediastinal cavity expands. Endo-abdominal or peritoneal pressure increases during an effort, especially when it is combined with forced expiration (Zatsiorskij and Sazonov[2], 1988). As a result of the internal support, pressure on intervertebral discs may be reduced by 40%; it is produced by the activity of the abdominal wall, intercostal, and diaphragm muscles.

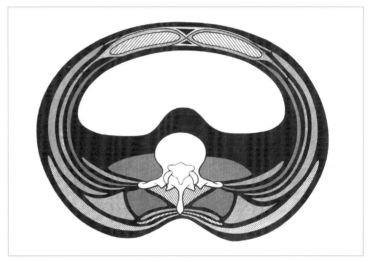

*The pelvis
(picture taken from Kapandji[3]).*

The picture of the pelvis (from Kapandji) reproduces a cutaway of the mediastinal cavity from which the action of the large muscles of the abdomen is evident: the external oblique, the internal oblique, and the transversus abdominis. These three muscles warp the abdominal cavity in three superimposed circles, joining at the front in a fibrous aponeurosis, into the weave in which the rectus abdominis is inserted. This already shows us that it is almost useless to work on the rectus abdominis to reduce the waistline because it doesn't have much influence. For this purpose we ought instead to focus on the three previously mentioned muscles. The abdominal fascia function as:

---

2 Zatsiorskij V.M. and Sazonov V.P. (1988). "Basi biomeccaniche nella prevenzione dei danni alla colonna lombare durante esercizio fisico - Revisione della bibliografia esistente", in *Atleticastudi*, 5.

3 Kapandji I.A (1983). *The Physiology of the Joints*, Elsevier Churchill Livingstone Publisher.

- **Stabilizers.**

Their role in containing the viscera and as stabilizers is ensured by isometric contractions which set the pelvis in an anatomic position. Let's think about it: If the erect posture is, or ought to be, the one most frequently adopted, our abdomen's number one function cannot be that of flexing the trunk on the ground, as with crunches and similar exercises, but rather it is the stabilization and rotation of the pelvis, working against gravity (does anyone do these exercises in gyms?).

- **Motors.**

The dynamic function is guaranteed by anisometric contractions of those muscles which allow flexion, lateral flexion, and rotation of the trunk and lifting of the pelvis. Once again we are not talking about one single muscle but about a functional, synergistic set. The majority of these movements still takes place in the upright position. If we think about trunk rotation, we realize that the first and most frequent gesture of this type happens when walking.

- **Respiratory mechanisms.**

The abdominal fascia contribute to expiration and, in particular, to forced expiration. The latter is produced by the activity of the abdominal wall muscles, the intercostal muscles, and the diaphragm. In many sports where there are expressions of strength and power, it is a virtually physiological activation.

The visual and aesthetic effects of good abdominal corset firmness, and specifically firmness of the transversus abdominis, are several.

The firmer the transversus abdominis, the thinner the waistline is, since there is an accent on the curve which delimits it laterally and which coincides with the area between the ribs and the pelvis: the hip line (hyperboloid line). A firm abdominal corset implies a series of benefits, the most important being:

- Less stress on the lumbar rachis.
- Greater core strength owing to the action of the pivot muscles.
- Reduction of back pains, owing to the increased stabilizing function.
- Reduced visceral ptosis.
- Improved synergy between lower and upper limbs in the work of kinematic chains.

7.6 THE CENTRIFUGE PRINCIPLE

In training theory, the core's importance is confirmed by its first-place ranking in the sequence of muscular areas to be trained in beginners: the centrifuge principle. This because the abdominal fascia and the joints which rely on it are the fulcrum upon which the forces coming from the upper body and the stress coming from the lower limbs (impact with the ground) are discharged. It is not by chance that the rachis is the area most subject to wear and to inflammatory pathologies: back pains, sciatica, and lumbago. And it is no less by chance that the back pains of 50-year-olds are becoming a heritage of the younger generations.

SCAPULOHUMERAL GIRDLE

8.1 PRESENTATION

Only functional training allows us to determine instances of contradictions in our locomotor apparatus.

The scapulohumeral joint is a case in point. It is an enarthrosis, like the coxofemoral joint. In other words, it has a greater range of movement compared to other joints.

Unlike the coxofemoral joint, however, where trunk weight contributes to the stabilization of the femur head within its articular cavity, in the scapulohumeral joint, the humerus is simply hanging from the trunk. In fact, when the deltoid muscle is at the point of maximum contraction with the arm abducted at 90 degrees, the humerus head deviates from the line of articular constraint.

The conformation of the shoulder joint tells us that our bodies' evolutionary choice has been one of mobility at the expense of stability.

The humerus head, in fact, only partially adheres to the glenoid cavity, remaining mostly outside the articular constraint.

Rather than entering the glenoid cavity, the humerus hangs from the trunk and moves in different directions. It is able to do this because of its active stability, created by the development of the nearby musculature, and its passive stability, ensured by the same muscles' tendons and by the ligaments.

Besides the scapula stabilizers, the only muscles with a prevailingly stabilizing function are those in the rotator cuff, a real articular reinforcement structure.

Question: Don't you find it strange that all the muscles richest in white fibers are inserted on the most unstable joint in the human body?

- Triceps long head: 67% of white fibers.
- Trapezius: 64% of white fibers.
- Latissimus dorsi and pectoralis muscle: 50-58% of white fibers.
- Deltoid (anterior, medial, posterior): 40% of white fibers, located chiefly in the anterior part.

Yet white fibers tell of high workloads, expressions of strength and power, and great tension. On a joint that is unstable? Almost as a confirmation of this, anyone who has trained the scapulohumeral girdle muscles intensely, though correctly and without overdoing it, has been virtually obliged to suffer through painful and inflammatory pain in this joint. Why such problems? Where do they stem from? Read the next paragraph, and you will find the answer.

8.2 ACTION OF THE SCAPULOHUMERAL GIRDLE

All the muscles involved in the movements of the shoulder region are distally inserted on the humerus, scapula, and clavicle. These three bone segments share everything.

TRAPEZIUS

The upper band plays an important role in all traction and lifting movements; it lifts the shoulder and rotates the scapula. The medial band retracts the shoulders, bringing them closer to the spine.

The lower band rotates the scapula and depresses the shoulder in synergy with the pectoralis minor muscle. Besides, when contracted unilaterally, the trapezius rotates the head laterally. We notice it when we have irritating neck problems, in which the contracture of the trapezius or the sternocleidomastoid heightens the pains associated with them.

DELTOID

This is a powerful abductor of the upper arm. It can raise the arm above the head. The clavicular bands lift the arm forward; the acromion bands lift it up laterally; and the scapular bands abduct the arm backward.

Besides, it has an active stabilizing role for the joint, which it covers like a cap.

It is activated in arm circumduction movements typical of swimming and boxing.

It works in synergy with the pectoralis major muscle in all pushing movements along different planes.

PECTORALIS MUSCLE

It works in synergy with the deltoid's clavicular bands in order to flex the shoulder at 90 degrees.

It adducts and intrarotates the shoulder, flexing the arm on the transverse plane.

With arms raised and fixed, it pulls the trunk upward (the climber's movement). In all suspension and support movements, it prevents the lowering of the trunk together with the latissimus dorsi. It is also active in the forward lifting of the arm from the outside back position (discus throw) and from the below back position (bowling). It cooperates in deep breathing. The synergy of the pectoralis with the triceps is extremely important in explosive, fast pushing movements (i.e., sweeping aside branches and twigs). The long head of the triceps is in fact statistically the muscle with the highest percentage of white fibers.

LATISSIMUS DORSI

It is dedicated to the extension, adduction, and internal rotation of the shoulder joint. In all suspension and support movements it contributes to the stabilization of the trunk. It forcefully lowers an elevated limb (e.g., in throwing or hitting movements). It also pulls the trunk toward the arms. As we can see, it performs many movements in synergy with the pectoralis, to which it is often and wrongly considered antagonist. (How can two muscles with the same distal insertion, both acting as intrarotators of the humerus, be antagonists?) When the hand is above the head, the latissimus dorsi pulls the arm down and backward against the resistance, as if we were lowering a portcullis. In a climbing action, the hand is placed above the head, and the latissimus dorsi works hard to pull the trunk toward the arms, lifting the whole body upward. In subjects with a functional lower-body functional deficit, if it is impossible to lift the body from a seated position by extending the lower legs, the hands can lean on the chair's armrests and push and lift the body up, exploiting the adduction action of the latissimus dorsi as it lifts the pelvis. When walking on crutches, the latissimus dorsi helps the hands bear the body's weight (see how monkeys walk).

SERRATUS ANTERIOR MUSCLE

Its action consists of pulling the scapula forward around the thorax (protraction). This movement increases the ability to stretch the upper limb forward, adding strength to the gesture of hitting with a fist or overcoming a resistance ahead (i.e., sweeping asides leaves and branches).

TRICEPS

This muscle has both biarticular and monoarticular features. Its long end, which is biarticular, acts as extensor of the forearm on the arm and as extensor of the arm on the trunk. It helps the pectoralis major and the deltoid in extensions and thrusts, and it helps the latissimus dorsi as it retracts and adducts the arm.

It is the antagonist of the biceps and the muscle responsible for the largest part of the arm's volume.

BRACHIAL BICEPS

This is another biarticular muscle. Can you then explain to me why I often see it trained with the elbows blocked alongside the trunk, with a monoarticular movement? The biceps' proximal segment is covered by the deltoid and the pectoralis major. The biceps is a flexor of the forearm and of the humerus; it is also a supinator of the forearm. When the elbow is extended, the biceps tenses to contrast the force of gravity. It also acts as a help to the latissimus dorsi in tractions.

8.3 FUNCTION OF THE SCAPULOHUMERAL GIRDLE

What is the function of the shoulder joints?

As we have seen, the scapulohumeral girdle is an extremely complex crossroad of muscles, tendons, articular systems, and a kinematic chain that is the victim of an apparent incongruity. Yet it is simple: The scapulohumeral girdle is a transducer of forces, a functional hub. Exactly like a rail hub, purpose of the shoulder joints is to transmit the forces coming from the lower body or the trunk to the upper body.

The scapulohumeral girdle's function suggests exercises and execution modes different from those used now and in the past. It tells us, for example, that there is a contraindication to training the deltoid with a load applied to the upper limb only (e.g., slow forward movement and slow barbells) without the help of the lower chains. It also tells us that we cannot ask for stability with excessive movement control and slow-motion executions from a joint that doesn't have this feature. It is better to train it with exercises in which the thrusting action starts from the lower body and, with their help, is then transmitted to the upper body via the scapulohumeral joint. Exercise examples include: push-press exercises with dumbbells or barbells and jerk, clean, and press exercises. Paradoxically, training requires much higher loads for a shorter timeframe. This is what this articular systems demands. Actually, if you think about it, any sporting activity featuring a transmission of forces from the lower to the upper part of the body, such as boxing, baseball, tennis, golf, weightlifting, or martial arts, follows this line. You will enjoy greater results in terms of strength and hypertrophy, and pains, inflammations, sub-acromion syndromes, and contrasting syndromes will decrease or even disappear.

8.4   GRIP TYPES

Grip is an issue which is seldom discussed in gyms. It is generally thought to be a factor of secondary importance. However, there comes a time in training when the subject starts adopting a personalized grip, often based on unorthodox suggestions (the most common is: "use this grip, you'll feel the pectoralis better"). Actually, strength stems from the grip. Power grips bring the maximum amount of the sensitive area of the fingers and the palm of the hand in contact with the object being gripped. The four fingers flex around the object while the thumb wraps around the opposite side; this way the sensitive receptors of the areas involved ensure there is the right pressure for controlling the barbell. In this action, all the muscles in the fingers and thumb that close the hand are active: the muscles of the thenar eminence and the hypothenar stabilize the palm's medial side against the object, the finger muscles grab, and the wrist extensors impart a stable base to the gripping action. Pay attention to when you close your fist; notice the hand, wrist, and forearm become one single functional block, a single segment. The harder the hand grips an object, the greater the wrist extensors' activity is and the more extensive the central nervous system's motor signal is. One of the primary reflexes in a newborn baby is flexing the fingers when pressure is exerted on the center of their palm. This kind of grip and the physiological reactions which subsequently intervene increases nerve response and muscular fibers recruitment.

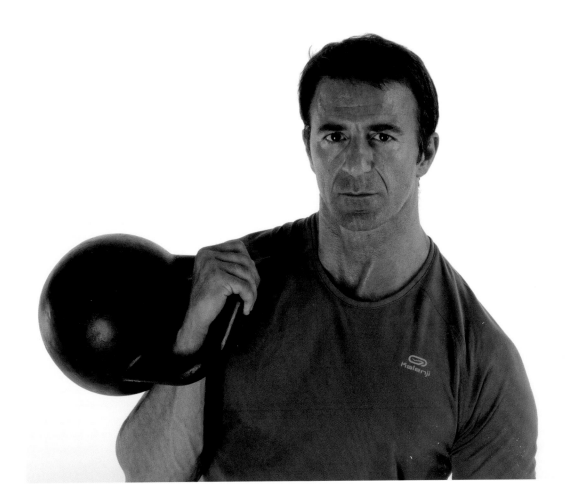

TIBIAL-TARSAL JOINT AND FOOT

9.1   PRESENTATION

The peculiarity of the foot is that it is the only part of the human body in continuous contact with the ground. While the vast majority of animals stand and ambulate on their fingers (digitigrade), man is a plantigrade (i.e., he or she rests the whole sole of the foot on the ground). When we stand, the ground exercises a force which is equal to and opposite to our body weight called ground reaction force. This and other forces are applied to the inferior limb joints—pelvis, knee, and ankles—which for this reason have a very high functional synergy. The role of the foot and ankle joints is:

- To orient the foot in order to set the sole correctly on the ground.
- To modify the shape and curvature of the plantar arch in order to adapt the foot to the ground's asperities and to create a system of shock absorbers between the ground and the leg.

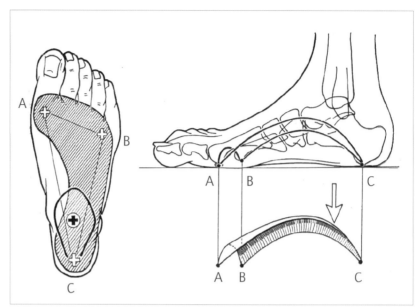

*The foot
(picture taken
from Kapandji[1]).*

---

1 Kapandji I.A (1983). *The Physiology of the Joints*, Elsevier Churchill Livingstone Publisher.

9.2 WALKING

In terms of the tibial-tarsal joint, the posterior tibial, gastrocnemius, and soleus are the muscles chiefly responsible for propulsion when walking, running, and jumping. The action of the calf muscles is augmented by arching the foot and flexing the toes. When the heel leaves the ground, the toes extend, increasing the plantar arch. Walking is technically like a fall cushioned by the contralateral limb. In ambulation, we have a foot-plant phase for approximately 60% of the stride and an oscillation phase, with the foot off the ground, for about 40%. This means there is an alternation of monopedal support and bipedal support phases. At the start of the foot-plant phase, the foot is forward of the trunk and pushes ahead and toward the ground, decelerating the body's fall and providing support. In the final phase, though, the foot is at the rear of the body and pushes down and backward, providing acceleration. Let me underline the intervention of the upper body in ensuring a correct, coordinated posture as a confirmation of our physiological conformation based on kinematic chains.

9.3 RUNNING

When running, the percentage ratios change drastically: the foot-plant phase ranges between 40 and 27%, depending on speed .The faster the athlete is, the shorter the ground foot-plant phase will be (sprinters reach about 22%).

Running efficiency is the result of the accumulation and release of potential energy within the elastic component of the tendons and of the energy-transfer action by the muscles that stretch across the lower joints. The kinematic chain activated by the running action sets off and involves initially both the gastrocnemius and the soleus. Both muscles help the action of the plantar arches and the forefoot. Then, in sequence, it involves the quadriceps, the hip extensor chain (femoral biceps and gluteus), and the abductors, compensating for the pelvis' fall at the foot plant. In terms of the foot, the action of the astragalus is essential. This is the bone that partitions the forces applied by the ankle and the tibia during the various phases. Because of the action of the plantar arches and the ligaments which run across the foot, the foot functions as a spring, ensuring the return of 80% of the elastic energy.

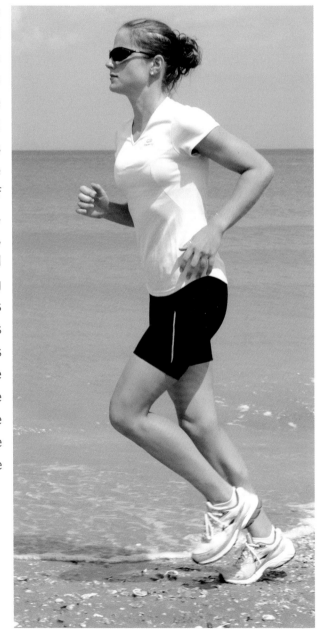

9.4   FOOT MOVEMENTS

As we have emphasized before, functional training points in one direction: training based on kinematic chains, following the evolutionary lines of the human race. It also suggests a different approach for gyms and sports centers: The action and function of a muscle, or a kinematic chain, should never be separated. We cannot disregard dynamic movements when training the musculature that runs across the tibial-tarsal joint, especially the triceps surae.

Let's think about it. These bone–joint structures have evolved for walking and running, and as such they have always been subjected to propulsive forces, both acceleration and deceleration. The exercises usually performed in gyms, even on machines, do not consider these features. It is a serious mistake to constrain our articular systems, which vary from individual to individual, by training only by the rectilinear path imposed by a machine. We have also seen how there is a synergy between the triceps surae and other muscles of the leg and thigh. It is obvious they have to be trained together in order to avoid a regression in terms of intra- and intermuscular coordination.

PART II – PERACTICE

10

BODY-WEIGHT EXERCISES

10.1   ORIGINS

The origins of body-weight exercises are very ancient. Instances of using body weight for exercising can be found in the Chinese, Egyptian, and Mycenaean cultures, as well as many others. Lycurgus maintained that in order to have better warriors more suited to the war effort, you had to start from athlete mothers, forged by physical exercise. Plutarch used the same expression when describing the customs of the Spartans, a famous warrior people. Galen, one of the fathers of medicine (131–201 AD), wrote in his work *De sanitate tuenda:*

"...This is what I consider as physical exercise or gymnastics, a term connected to the gymnasium, where people go to anoint themselves, enjoy a massage, engage in wrestling, discus throwing, or in other sporting activities."

More than one thousand years after that, Mercurial recommended discus throwing, rope climbing, race walking, mountain climbing, and long jump as the activities that gave the most benefits. In those days, sportsmen and athletes used to train standing up; benches and machines didn't exists, only more or less rudimentary weights, medicine balls, dumbbells, rocks, the trapeze, ropes, and still rings.

There was no theoretical basis to training. An athlete had to be strong, fast, and tough. And he became all of these things.

10.2   PRESENTATION

Our body is the tool, the starting and finishing line of functional training. As Michael Boyle (2010), the father of American functional training, says, "We will never be good at managing an external weight (barbell, dumbbell or other) if first we aren't good at managing our own body." Train the body to move by acquiring efficiency and awareness: This is the objective.

10.2.1   Load types

When we do body-weight exercises, there are essentially four types of load we can use:

1. Body weight as resistance.
2. The weight of the falling body as resistance (e.g., downward jumps, obstacle jumping, upward jumps).
3. Ordinary loads, such as dumbbells and barbells.
4. Unconventional loads, such as kettlebells, sandbags, and medicine balls.

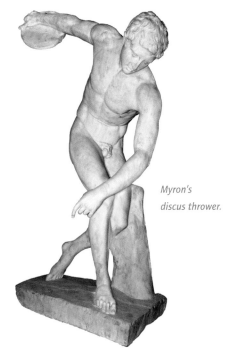

Myron's discus thrower.

The first type, using body weight as resistance, will be our priority. We will rediscover our body— our first tool and one we often forget about. As a first approach to training, you should work on body and movement awareness with exercises that are almost exclusively body weight. Anyone who says that body-weight exercises are easy simply doesn't know them. Gymnasts work with body-weight exercises, and their physique and athletic expressions are very stunning. Starting out with a squat to train the legs without having first tested and trained the kinematic chains involved through a free-standing leg flexion exercise is like building a house without a foundation. Work and train with body-weight exercises. You will never regret it.

10.3   TRAINING RULES

Before we begin the practical part, we need to outline a few rules.

1. **Outfit.** Wear comfortable clothes that leave you free to move without constraints or excessive compression.

2. **Shoes.** No other type of sports shoe has developed technically like the running shoe. This is logical, isn't it? Because we have to use them to do thousands of steps, we must put the best technique to the service of the feet and their support structures. But especially for the less demanding exercises, at least in terms of the joints, go back to your roots and train barefoot. Let's not forget that we were born barefoot, and we have evolved barefoot, too. Someone has raised the objection that going sole-less we are more vulnerable to injuries and articular trauma. The objection is not valid. We do have a physiological sole, the calcaneal fat pad, which covers the whole foot sole with an increased thickness beneath the heel and the metatarsal heads. Besides, proprioception—the key to smart movement—begins with work done with a barefoot sole.

3. **Mental attitude.** Take your training seriously. It isn't a matter of time; studies say that training twice a week is enough to yield results. Devote those 30-50 min to training your body intensely and with concentration and a will to improve. Remember that there is a level of intensity below which there will be no biological modifications in your muscles and endogenous systems. You will have only wasted your time.

4. **Practice.** Practice doesn't make perfect. Perfect practice makes perfect. Try every exercise many times, repeat it in front of other coaches, and even do it with your eyes closed (the Soviet school suggests this solution, too). You will have to feel it; the exercise must be inside you.

5. **Execution.** Take no prisoners with execution. Let me explain. Many times in gyms I see exercises performed with bounces, back thrusts, and other stuff, the person going to any length to add an extra repetition. You must be aware that with this kind of execution you are training your ego, not your muscles or your muscular chains in a way that is appropriate. What is the use of teaching a bar traction for the latissimus dorsi if you then teach your students to cheat using back thrusts?

6. **Exhaustion.** Reach exhaustion: yours, not that of the partner helping you! Be objective.

7. **Balanced training.** Always give priority to the frontal part of the body, especially the trunk and the upper limbs. When stuck in a routine, every Monday, it's nothing but the horizontal bench! Isn't it time to change? Consider that, by and large, the things you least like doing in the gym are those that are most useful (e.g., squats, walking lunges, abdominal exercises).

8. **Training diary.** Keeping a daily training diary may seem maniacal, and perhaps it is. But do keep a note-book to mark down your objectives and the progress you make in this direction.

10.4 LOWER-BODY EXERCISES

FRONT SQUAT

Starting position

- **A** | Stand and hold a barbell firmly. The wrists are broken (i.e., the hands are back with the palms facing up), the hands resting on the clavicles, the elbows high and pointing forward.

Execution

- **B** | Bend the legs and sit back into a full squat.

  Keep the elbows high.

  Aim for the deepest possible movement, maintaining the spine's physiological curves.

  Return to the starting position.

  Complete the required number of repetitions.

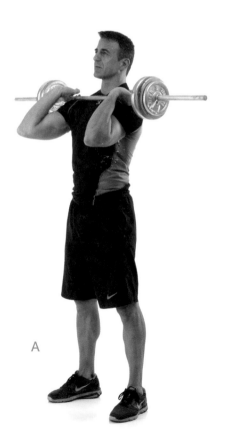

A

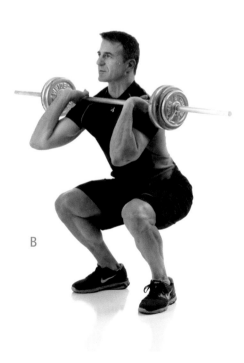

B

Discussion

I know, I talk about body-weight exercises, and I start with the frontal squat. This is meant as a reminder. This is the most neglected and undervalued exercise in gyms and in fitness training. Wrongly so! Many people begin with a classic squat without being ready for it, both technically and in terms of the coordination and fluidity of the kinematic and articular chains involved. The front squat not only teaches the correct squat technique—it is a natural preparation for it—but also, compared to its more famous cousin exercise, it features:

■ fewer difficulties with the stance;

■ a better load and body-weight distribution;

■ a deeper movement, translating into a greater activation of the gluteus;

■ a smaller load on the lower back;

■ excellent stimulation of the erector spinae, the multifidus, the longissimus dorsi, the sacral-lumbar, and the quadratus lumborum muscles; and

■ involvement of the rectus abdominis and the core muscle in an excellent stabilizing action.

Personally, I believe this is one of the best preventive, and even treatment, exercises for chronic lumbago, based on empirical tests with athletes. I will also admit that I consider it a treatment for acute lumbago as well, when used with core exercises that use fitness balls. This is a personal opinion, of course, but if experience counts for anything, the effects of this exercise go well beyond its appearance. Besides, it activates the gluteus to a greater degree, and this is an element much sought after by women as an objective for every training program. So this exercise is a must for anyone.

LEG FLEXION

Starting position

- A | Stand with your legs at shoulder width. Extend the arms in front of you in a neutral position (i.e., thumbs upward); the scapulae must be adducted.

Execution

- B | Bend the legs and sit back in a controlled fashion until you reach a full squat.
  Extending the legs return to the starting position.
  Complete the required number of repetitions.

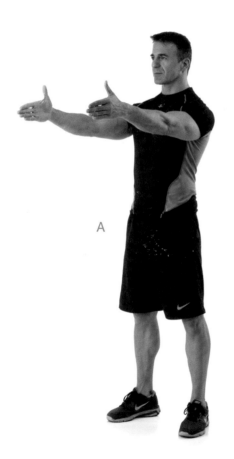

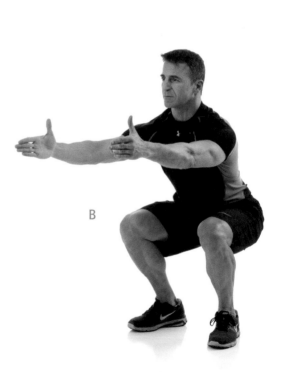

Discussion

Discussing squats would require a whole book. In the history of athletics, there isn't a training technique which has been analyzed more, instant by instant, moment by moment, with all its implications. Let's examine the most important ones:

- *Position of the scapulae:* they are adducted in order to keep the upper back in correct position; the trapezius and the latissimus dorsi are essential for correct upper-body and spine posture.
- *Spine:* it is in the neutral position; performing the exercise with the greatest possible movement range must not prevent you from maintaining the spine's natural curves.
- *Movement:* squat as deep as possible, taking care of what is noted in the previous points. Electromyographic studies tell us that the deeper the squat is, the more the gluteus maximus is activated and stimulated.

Look around gyms, and you will see that maybe, and I repeat, maybe, 1 person in 20 is performing a passable squat. The squat is a fundamental exercise for a total-body motor activation and for the physiological responses it generates. It is primarily important for generating the hormonal response. A training program without squats is like the opera *Turandot:* an incomplete work.

ASYMMETRIC SQUAT

Starting position

- **A** | Stand with the legs at shoulder width. Extend the arms in front of you in a neutral position (thumbs upward); the scapulae must be adducted.
  Bring the right foot 4-6 in. (10-15 cm) forward of the left foot.

Execution

- **B** | Bend the legs and sit back in a controlled fashion until you reach a full squat.
  Rise up again and complete the number of repetitions required.
  Invert the position of your limbs and execute this exercise again with the same number of repetitions.

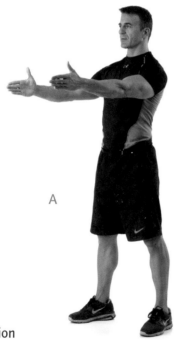

A

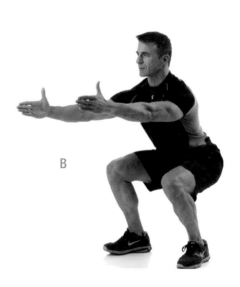

B

Discussion

This specific exercise was taught to me by Michael Boyle[1] (2010) in Los Angeles, with the following explanation: Do we ever, in daily and in sporting life, find ourselves executing squats or other frontal plane flexion with limbs perfectly aligned? Let's try to work asymmetrically and see the effect it has. It is interesting to feel how the perception of the exercise and of the muscles that are stimulated changes by varying one foot's position just a little. Specifically, the adductor and the gluteus minimus and medius of the contralateral leg work harder. A fine exercise and excellent preparation.

1 Boyle M. (2010). Personal communication, *Perform Better Convention*, LA.

SQUAT JUMP

Starting position

- **A |** Stand with the legs at shoulder width. Extend the arms in front of you in a neutral position (thumbs upward); the scapulae must be adducted.

Execution

- **B |** Bend the legs and sit back in a controlled fashion until you reach a full squat.

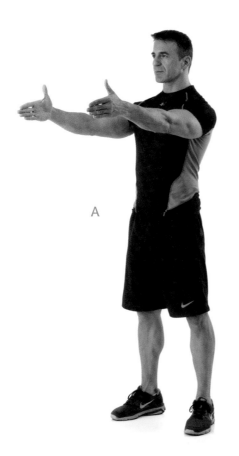

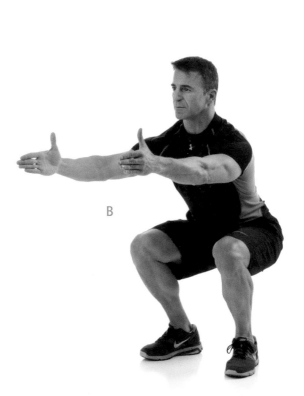

- **C|** From here, jump explosively upward, using the arms to help with the movement.

- **D |** Cushion the landing phase with your legs. Take a second to stabilize your position, and then complete your repetitions.

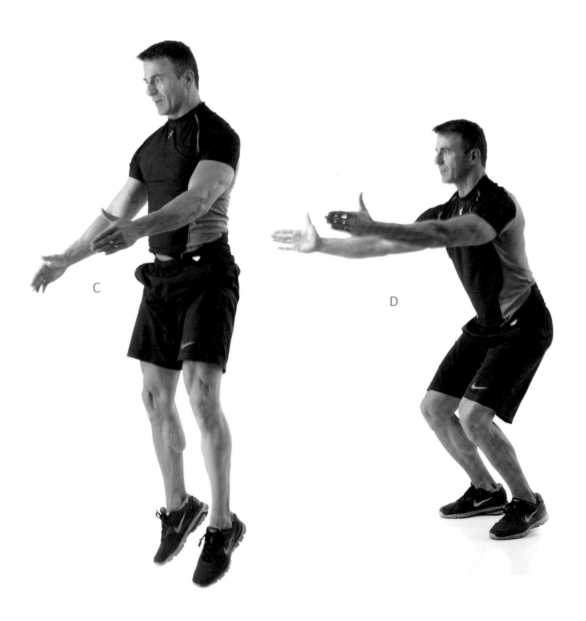

C

D

Discussion

The same argument given initially for the squat is valid for the squat jump, at least partly. According to many, the squat jump is equivalent to a direct route to back ache, especially with the addition of a load, such as a barbell. Much could be said on the use of this exercise. In fact, when the loaded barbell is positioned at the level of the trapezius, its downward acceleration (not excluding body weight) applies stress on the rachis and the joints of the lower limbs. Yet all coaches will use it at some stage in the season. There is a reason for this: It is a functional exercise, because the hip extensor chain works both in its action, flexion–extension, and its function, propulsion. This exercise is effective for any expression of explosive strength and speed strength. Now some advice:

1. Start teaching the squat movement the correct way, beginning with the free-standing exercise.
2. Work with preliminary or preparatory exercises on all the kinematic chains involved (e.g., wall squats or overhead squats, which we shall soon see). Yes, work the lower limbs, but also work the spine and back extensor muscles (quadratus lumborum, erector spinae, longissimus dorsi, semispinalis dorsi, and multifidus).
3. If you are using a lighter load (a light barbell or dumbbells), position the equipment forward, as in the front squat, keeping the elbows high. You will thus reduce the load incidence on the lower back.
4. Absorb as best you can the load on the joints of the lower limbs, cushioning it. And take a second to stabilize your position. I recommend no more than five repetitions per set, given the tendon and ligament stress to which the joints involved in this exercise are subjected.

OVERHEAD SQUAT

Starting position

- **A |** Stand with the legs at shoulder width. Raise your arms upward, close to the head.

Execution

- **B |** Bend the legs and sit back to a full squat.
  While you bend, extend the arms backward to keep them high and perpendicular above you.
  Return to the starting position.

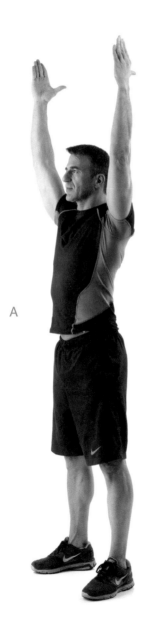

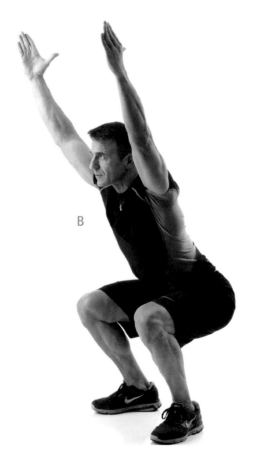

Discussion

I have always had a weakness for overhead squats; they are little-known but outstanding exercises. They require control and balance. Thanks to the long lever, overhead squats activate the parascapular and paravertebral musculatures and the humerus retractor muscles (trapezius, cuff extrarotators, rhomboid), leading to significant postural improvements. These exercises are essential to prepare the body for the heavier basic exercises. Of course this isn't an easy exercise, at least for beginners. For this reason, the preparation and the difficulty progression are very important.

- *First step:* Start with an ordinary flexion of the legs. Once you have reached a full squat, raise one arm upward with a slight rotation of the trunk to accommodate for the raised arm, then return to the standing position.
- *Second step:* Execute a squat in which only one arm is raised from beginning to end.

Now you can do the full exercise. During the first two executions, you will be surprised when feeling the activation of the oblique muscles. The next step will of course be working with a barbell, kettlebell, or sandbag overhead.

PRISONER SQUAT

Starting position

- **A |** Stand with the legs at shoulder width. Cross your hands behind your head; the scapulae are adducted and the elbows spread wide.

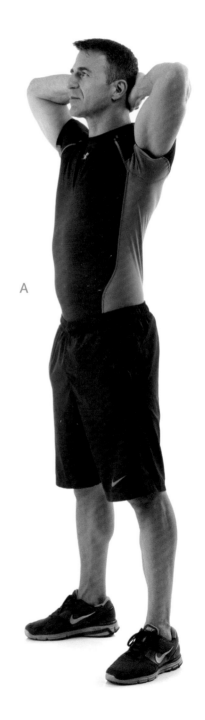

A

Execution

- **B |** Bend the legs in a controlled fashion and sit back into a full squat.
  As you bend down, emphasize the abduction of the elbows.
  Rise up again and complete the repetitions.

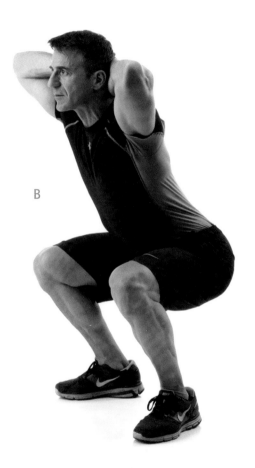

B

Discussion

The position of the upper body activates the parascapular musculature and the back's extensor chain. Also, the arms act as a balancing system, and without their help, the core and the whole abdominal fascia are stimulated to a greater degree. Add the work on the lower body, and there you have it. This is an excellent exercise with a great postural value. Its progression allows for the execution of increasingly complex variations—even monopedal ones—always in the prisoner position.

ONE-LEG SQUAT

Starting position

- **A |** Stand and raise the right leg, then extend it slightly backward and flex it.
  The arms are along the sides for coordination and to compensate a possible (and common) loss of balance.

Execution

- **B |** Bend the legs and sit back in a controlled fashion until you reach an almost full squat—or a full one, if your articular mobility allows it—leaning slightly forward with your body.
  Rise slowly, without placing the right leg on the ground.
  Stabilize your position and start again.
  Complete the required number of repetitions, then repeat with the other leg.

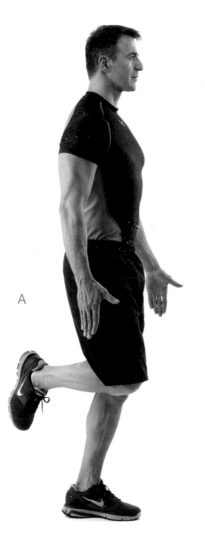

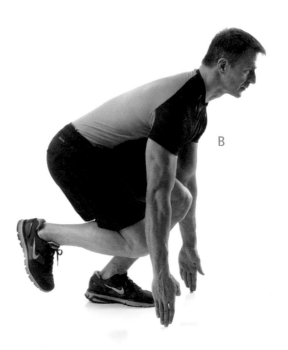

Discussion

In my opinion this is absolutely the best glutes and thighs exercise, including free-standing ones. The entire body load, or at least a good 80% of it, is applied to the whole hip extensor chain. With just a few controlled repetitions, you will feel the gluteus and the quadriceps working as you never have before. Also, it trains proprioception—perhaps the most important athletic ability—coordination, and balance as few other exercises do. As a measure or check for the depth of the squat, you should touch the ground with at least your fingertips. The one-leg squat and all its variations (pistol squat, one-leg squat jump; one-leg burpees) is a virtually mandatory exercise when we consider athletic strengthening. It also offers ample opportunities for progression, from adding a jump in the squat phase (one-leg squat jump) to an increased load via a sandbag (resting sandbag on shoulder during one-leg squat), or medicine ball. After the strength-training phase with Olympic and basic exercises in the gym, monolateral work is a must, at least for elite athletes. Rugby, combat sports, judo, martial arts, volleyball, football, basketball—no sport can ignore this exercise. Even from a fitness point of view, it takes the podium as one of the most effective exercises in producing Brazilian glutes.

WALL SQUAT

Starting Position

- **A |** Stand with you back against a wall. Spread your feet apart to shoulder width, the toes touching the wall.

Execution

- **B |** Open your arms to the sides of the trunk, parallel to the ground.
- **C |** Start bending your legs and sit back in

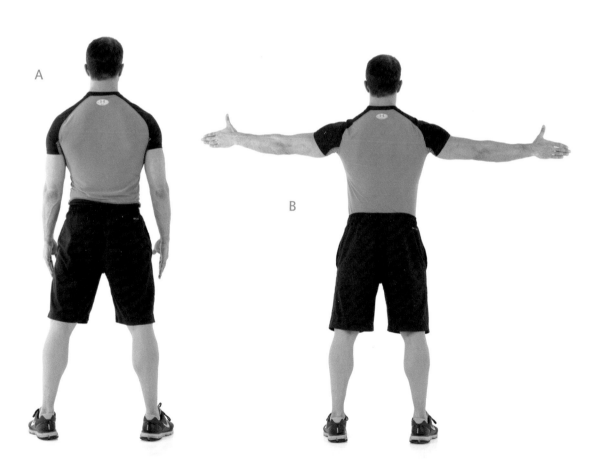

a controlled fashion into a squat. Push the coxofemoral joint out by flexing it and lean forward with your chest to compensate. Sink as low as you can into the squat (stop when you feel you are losing balance), then rise up again.

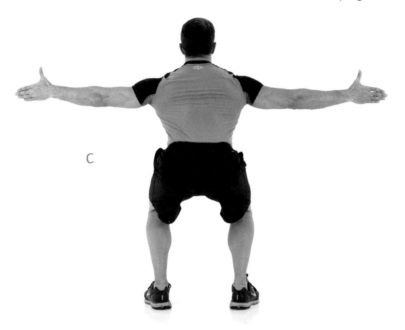

C

Discussion

This is a wonderful exercise, brought back to the fore by Pavel Tsatsouline. It is a fantastic preliminary and preparatory exercise for heavy squats. It increases the functionality of the hip joint and the activation of the hamstring muscles and femoral group. It significantly stimulates and reinforces the paravertebral musculature, especially at the lumbar-hinge level. Also, given the position of the arms, the humerus retractor muscles and parascapular muscles are under stress, too. This is a must for any athletic training, at least in the initial stages. The first objectives for any coach, personal trainer, or instructor must be to strengthen the weak links in the kinematic chains. This is just the exercise to do that.

LUNGE–BEND–LUNGE–BEND (LU.BE.LU.BE.)

Starting position

- **A |** Stand with the legs together.

Execution

The acronym Lu.Be.Lu.Be. indicates a sequence of movements: lunge backward-bend-lunge forward-bend. So:

- **B |** Move your right leg back (on the sagittal plane) to perform a backward lunge.

- **C |** Bring the right leg level with the left leg (on the frontal plane), keeping them separate at shoulder width, and execute a squat.

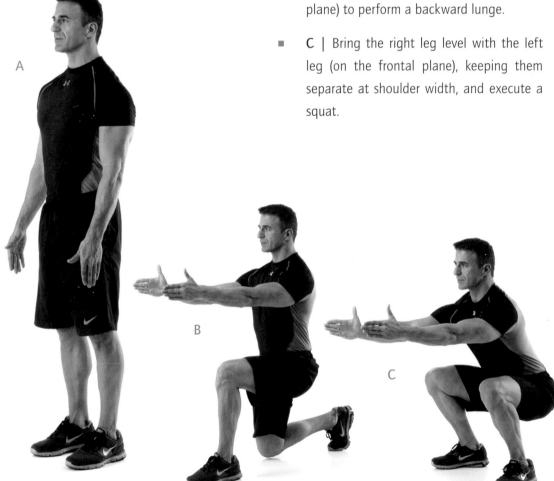

■ **D |** Bring the right leg forward and perform a forward lunge.

■ **E |** Bring the right leg close to the left leg and flex them with legs and feet together, descending into a squat while the heels remain touching with the ground. Repeat the sequence with the left leg. Complete the required number of repetitions.

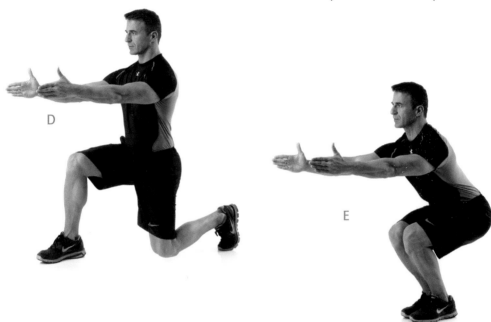

Discussion

I created this exercise thinking about the features of the hip joint, the coxofemoral joint. It is an enarthrosis—a very mobile joint (the most mobile after the upper-back joints)—with several movement planes. Why limit ourselves to exercises on only the frontal or sagittal planes (i.e., squats or lunges)? Why not train the muscles which insert into the hip with one single exercise, working on several planes? You can feel the difference: The quadriceps, gluteus, adductors (very much so!), and abductors all take part in this fantastic mix of movements. It is often said, wrongly so, that body-weight exercises are lighter. Well, I will take a wager on this exercise. Perform sets of 4 circuits per leg, alternating the legs, and let me know. And you have worked with body weight only! Try to do it with two dumbbells, even light ones. This is undoubtedly an excellent choice for athletic training, as well as for toning programs and circuit training.

WALKING LUNGE

Starting position

- A | Stand with legs together.

Execution

- B | Take a step forward with the left leg. You will find yourself in the lunge position (the starting position for lunges).

- C | Kneel down until the right knee is brushing the ground.

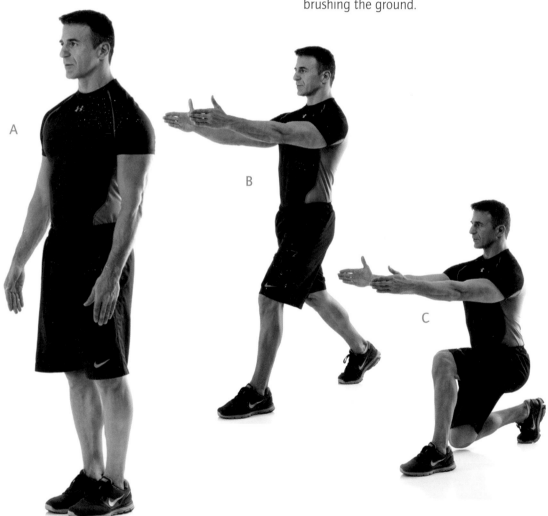

■ **D** | From this position, with one single step, bring the right leg forward and up.

■ **E** | Kneel down until the left knee is brushing the ground. Perform the required number of repetitions.

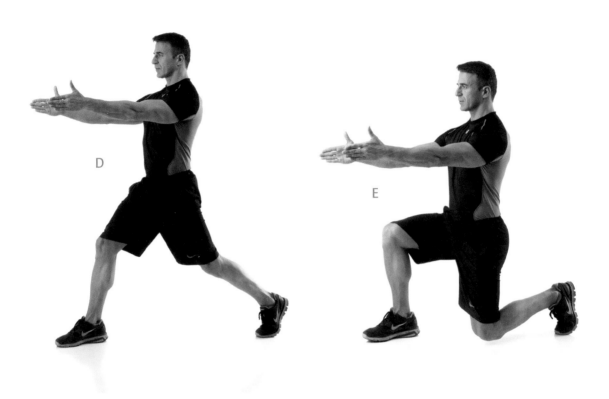

Discussion

This is functional training *par excellence*. We have action and function of the gluteus and the hip extensor muscles in one single exercise. The walking lunge has everything. It activates the hip and pelvis stabilizers, the adductors, and the abdominal fascia and the trunk stabilizer muscles with evident improvements in posture. It works on balance, coordination, and proprioception. And yet in gyms it is wholly ignored by men, who prefer performing the same movement when stationary or alternating the position of the legs. These are good exercises, even as a preparation for the walking lunge, but they are no match for it in terms of effectiveness. Why? Let me reveal this unmentionable taboo: This is a tough exercise. Very tough. And it doesn't even offer the satisfaction of a heavy load. So it is too much for the self-esteem of those who think that a heavy load is the thing when training, and who cares if a wrong execution cancels out the results. And yet the walking lunge works, like few other exercises do.

WALKING LUNGE WITH ROTATION

Starting position

- **A |** Stand with legs together, then extend the arms forward and interlock the hands. The abdominal fascia is slightly contracted, and the scapulae are adducted.

Execution

B | Take a step forward with the right leg and at the same time:

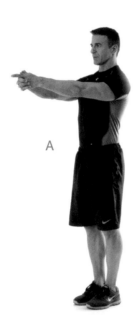

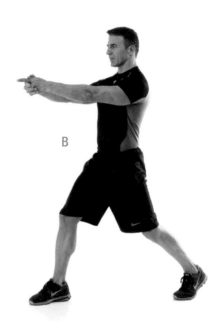

Discussion

This is an evolution of the previous exercise, so it is definitely functional! Summary of the previous exercise: It is a great exercise for the gluteus, femoral, quadriceps, and adductor muscles. The different position the upper body adopts during the movement influences and modifies the activation of the kinematic chains involved. In this case you will feel a greater stimulus to the abdominal fascia, particularly the large muscles of the abdomen: the interior obliques, exterior obliques, and transversus muscles. The rectus abdominis participates chiefly with a stabilizing function, as antagonist of the quadratus lumborum, in order to prevent an excessive load on the lumbar spine. Let me remind you that trunk rotations and any movement on the transverse plane are key components in nearly all performance sports. Exercises which involve several different planes are extremely effective for building

- **C** | 1. Bend the left leg until you brush the ground with your knee in a half-kneel position; 2. contract the abdomen and, keeping the arms straight in front of you, rotate the trunk toward the forward leg (in this case, the right leg).

- **D** | From this position, take a step forward with the left leg.

- **E** | At the same time, lower your right knee into a half-squat, and rotate the trunk to the left. Complete the required number of repetitions.

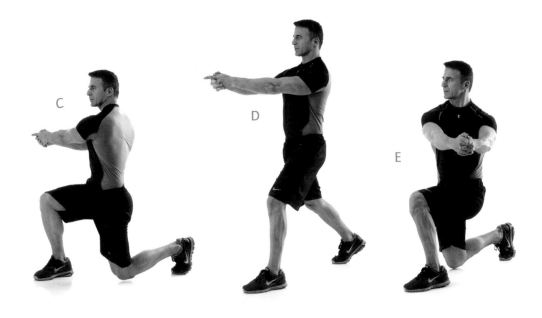

a complete athlete. This exercise can also be performed with a contrary rotation of the trunk (i.e., rotating it to the right and back, while bringing the left leg forward). In this case you will feel a greater stretching of the oblique muscles and the rectus femoris in the eccentric phase. Important: The joint activation of the lower body on the sagittal plane and the trunk and the upper body on the transverse plane destabilizes the whole body. Destabilizing exercises are always included, sometimes excessively so, in athletic training. You will often see exercises performed on unstable surfaces, such as Bosu balls, exercise balls, or proprioception boards. Because destabilization also follows its own progression, this isn't always the right choice. As a first step, do not perform an exercise on an unstable base (we were not born on *Avatar's* flying islands, but on solid ground!). Do it with an asymmetric or mobile load to create instability. You should work with an unstable base at a later stage.

WALKING LUNGE AND FLEX

Starting position

■ **A |** Stand with legs and feet together, then extend the arms above your head and interlock the hands. The abdominal fascia is slightly contracted (imagine you are bringing the ribs closer to the pelvis).

Execution

■ **B |** Take a step forward with the right leg.

■ **C |** At the same time: 1. bend the left knee in a half-squat; 2. flex the trunk laterally toward the forward leg (in this case, the right leg).

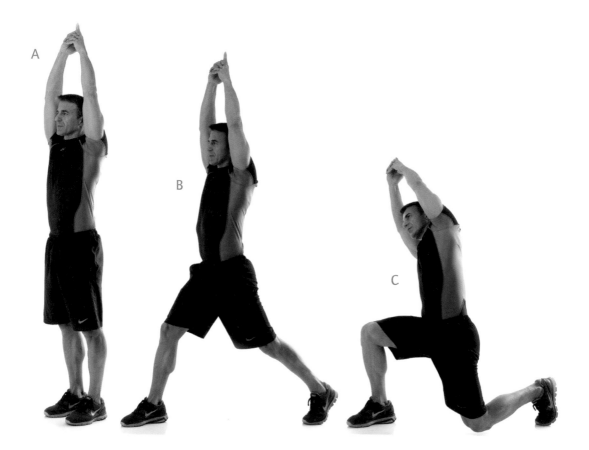

■ **D** | From this position, bring the left leg forward.

■ **E** | At the same time, lower the right knee and flex the trunk to the left. Complete the required number of repetitions.

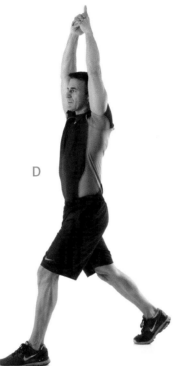

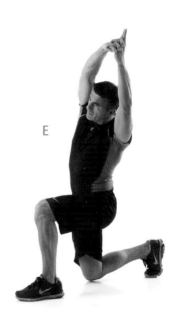

Discussion

What we said about the previous exercise holds true: It is excellent for the gluteus, femoral, adductor, and quadriceps muscles. The position which the upper body adopts during the exercise calls upon different kinematic chains; you will feel a greater engagement of the abdominal fascia, especially the interior and exterior oblique muscles. Here, too, the rectus abdominis intervenes with a stabilizing action, preserving the trunk from excessive extension and tilting. Also, the paravertebral and humerus retractor muscles—the parascapular muscles, the cuff extrarotators, the trapezius, and the posterior deltoid—are all stimulated. This chain's firmness guarantees a better and more correct posture. This exercise can also be performed with a reverse movement of the trunk (i.e., flexing to the right while bringing the left leg forward). In this case you will feel a greater stretching of both the oblique muscles and the rectus femoris of the back leg in the eccentric phase. This is an exercise you should practice and work on. It is excellent for proprioception, too, seeing as how it progressively introduces destabilization.

PRISONER WALKING LUNGE

Starting position

- **A |** Stand with legs together, hands interlocked behind the head; the scapulae are adducted.

Execution

- **B |** Take a step forward with the left leg and lower the right knee into a half-squat in a controlled fashion until it brushes the ground.

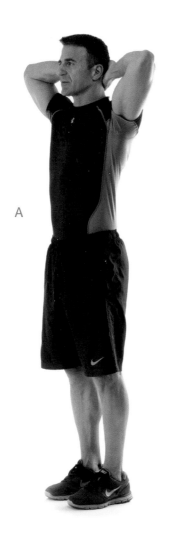

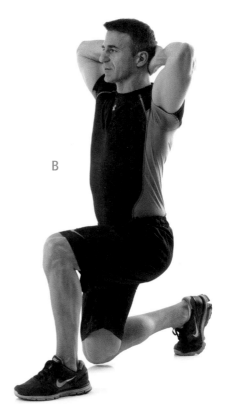

■ **C** | Rise again.

■ **D** | Take a step forward with the right leg and lower the left knee. Return to the starting position and continue with the required number of repetitions.

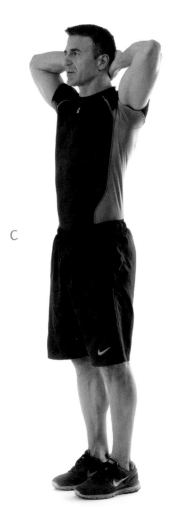

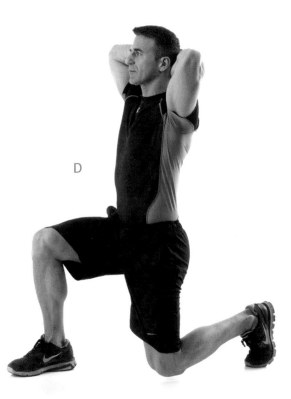

Discussion

This exercise works on the gluteus, femoral, adductor, and quadriceps muscles as well as the abdominal fascia. The position of the upper body activates the parascapular musculature and the back's extensor chain. Besides, executing the walking lunge without the help of the upper body for coordination and balance increases the activation of the abdominal fascia in order to lend stability to the trunk. It also trains proprioception, coordination, and balance. It is an excellent functional exercise with a postural value. Remember, the body should be a well-fitting outfit: This is our objective.

MONSTER LUNGE WITH ELBOW IN

Starting position

- **A** | Stand with legs together, hands interlocked behind the head; the scapulae are adducted.

Execution

- **B** | Raise the right leg, flexing the contralateral thigh.

- **C** | Extend the right leg.

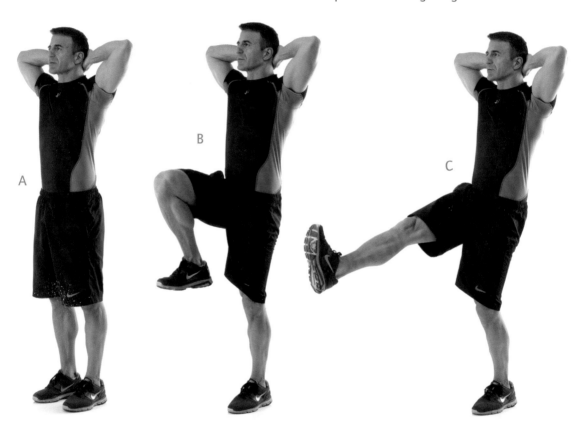

Discussion

I love this exercise. And I am loved back, I think, seeing I am one of its greatest promoters. In one word, it is comprehensive, besides the fact that it subjects the body to total-body training. The position of the upper body activates the parascapular musculature and the back's extensor chain, visibly affecting posture in a short time. The walking phase, split in flexion, extension, and alternate forward movement of the limbs, requires significant control, coordination, and proprioception.

- **D |** Take a step forward.

- **E |** At the same time, 1. lower the left knee; 2. rotate the trunk, and flex the torso forward and laterally down, bringing the right elbow inside the right thigh, level with the knee.

- **F |** Now, flexing the left thigh and leg, lift up again from the half-squat position. Repeat the movement on the other side, completing the required number of repetitions.

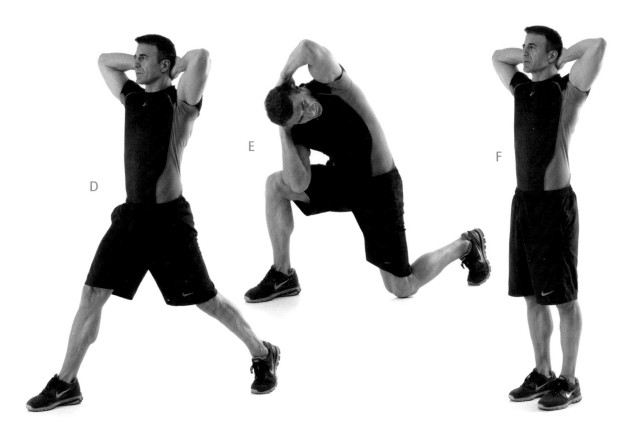

Lunging without the help of the upper body for coordination and balance increases the activation of the entire abdominal fascia. This stabilizes the trunk and also trains proprioception. The lateral flexion of the torso fully stimulates the oblique muscles. During the rising leg forward-flexion phase, the rectus abdominis works as well. This is an excellent functional exercise with a postural value.

MONSTER LUNGE WITH ELBOW OUT

Starting position

- **A** | Stand with legs together, hands interlocked behind the head; the scapulae are adducted.

Execution

- **B** | Raise the right leg, flexing the ipsilateral thigh.

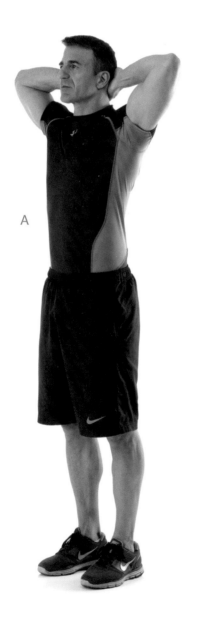

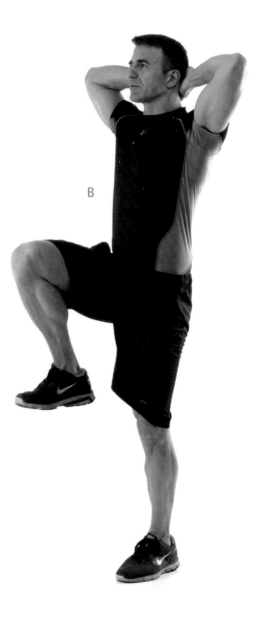

- **C |** Extend the right leg.

- **D |** Take a step forward.

- **E |** At the same time, 1. lower the left knee; 2. rotate and flex the torso to the right, bringing the left elbow outside the right thigh.

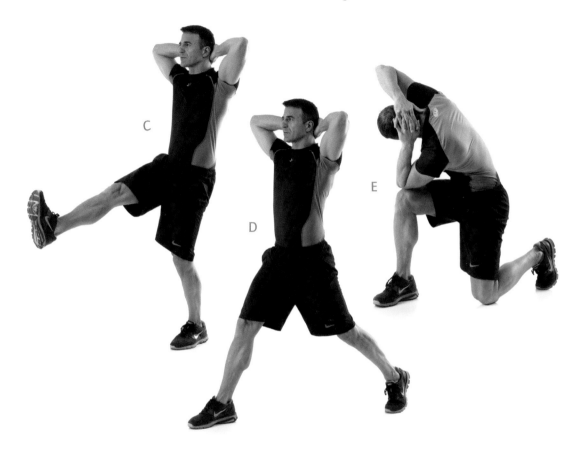

Discussion

This is very similar to the previous exercise, at least with regards to the work of the lower body. The position of the upper body activates the parascapular musculature and the back's extensor chain. The walking phase, split into flexion, extension, and alternate forward movement of the limbs, requires great control and significant coordination. Lunging without the help of the upper body for coordination and balance increases the activation of the abdominal fascia. This stabilizes the trunk and also trains proprioception. The rotation of the torso works synergistically on the interior obliques and the contralateral exterior oblique muscles. This is an excellent functional and postural exercise.

CRAB

Starting position

- **A** | From the squat's crouching position, place legs slightly wider than shoulder width and extend the arms forward, keeping the palms turned inward.

Execution

Keep the pelvis low and imitate a crab's lateral walk.

- **B** | Move the left leg inward quickly by about 8-12 in. (20-30 cm).

- **C** | Then immediately afterward, move the right leg outward. Complete the number of steps required and repeat in the opposite direction.

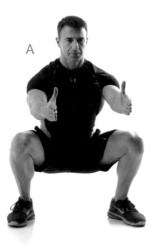

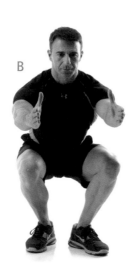

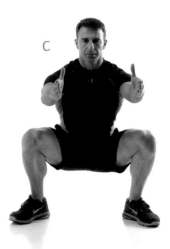

Discussion

The squat position is widely used in contact sports, like rugby, American football, judo, wrestling, sumo, mixed martial arts (MMA), and others. This exercise trains all the chains involved as well as the skills required. The quadriceps, adductors, gluteus muscles, and the entire abdominal fascia are thoroughly tested; specifically, the quadriceps work virtually isometrically, while the adductors work as hip stabilizers. The lactacid component is very high, especially if you do timed work. The objective is to remain in the squat position during the lateral shift without oscillating the pelvis up and down. This is a good exercise.

OVERHEAD CRAB

Starting position

- **A |** From the squat's crouching position with the legs slightly wider than shoulder width, extend the arms overhead, keeping the palms turned inward.

Execution

Keep the pelvis low and imitate a crab's lateral walk.

- **B |** Move the left leg inward quickly by about 8-12 in. (20-30 cm).

- **C |** Then immediately afterward, move the right leg outward.
  Complete the required number of steps and repeat in the opposite direction.

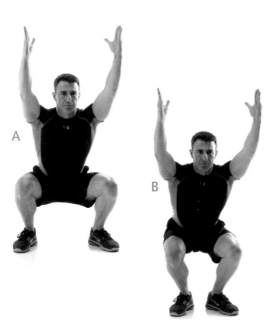

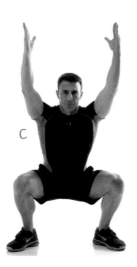

Discussion

These overhead exercises are brilliant and almost unknown in gyms. Posture and position aren't enough to explain the impact they have on the body in terms of the nerve and the musculoskeletal systems. As mentioned, the squat position is widely used in contact sports, like rugby and American football but also judo, wrestling, sumo, MMA, and others. The quadriceps, adductors, gluteus muscles, and the entire abdominal fascia are thoroughly tested. The lactacid component is very high, especially if you do timed work. The position of both arms, as they extend overhead, stimulates the whole paravertebral and parascapular musculature as well as the humerus retractor muscles, improving posture significantly. The objective is of course to remain in the squat position while executing the exercise without oscillating the pelvis up and down.

SURF LUNGE

Starting position

- **A |** Stand and take a step forward with the right leg; the arms are open laterally to facilitate balance.

  Raise the left heel and the right forefoot so that only the right heel and the tip of the left foot are touching the ground.

Execution

- **B |** Lower the left knee to the half-kneeling position.

  Rise up again and complete the required number of repetitions.

  Repeat the exercise with the left leg forward.

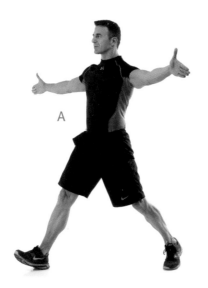
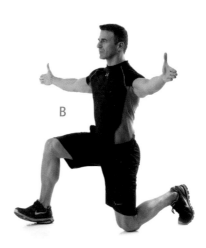

Discussion

I created this exercise for a competitive surfer, including it in the pre-racing part of his or her athletic training. Only afterward I realized how valuable it could be for other sports which engage balance, proprioception, and pivot muscles; not excluding the whole extensor and stabilizer musculature of the hip and leg: the tibial and peroneal muscles, the calves, femoral, quadriceps, adductor, and gluteus muscles. Given the destabilized position, abdominal fascia work is important, too. The whole core is involved in every phases of the exercise. Compared to normal lunges, the interesting element in this exercise is that different kinematic chains are engaged, or at any rate they are engaged differently, which is something. This exercise will be a significant benchmark for sports in which such synergies are important, such as skating, rhythmic gymnastics, ice or rink hockey, and surfing.

BACKWARD LUNGE

Starting position

- **A |** Stand with the legs together. The arms are alongside the body, the palms of the hands facing forward.

Execution

- **B |** Move the right leg back, following a diagonal outward trajectory.

- **C |** Flex the leg, lowering the right knee. From this position, take another step backward with the left leg, lowering the ipsilateral knee. Complete the required repetitions.

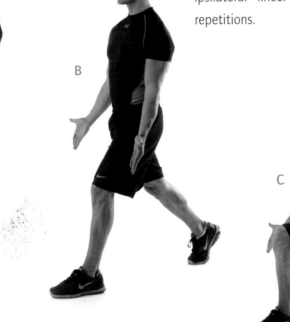

Discussion

All the exercises that involve a backward movement require a degree of control, coordination, and balance markedly superior to those necessary for forward movements. The reason is simple: Our first control system, sight, is missing. Besides that of the hip extensor chain—gluteus, femoral, and quadriceps muscles—the involvement of the adductors group is interesting, both as hip stabilizers and actively as flexors and extensors, according to the position of the contralateral limb. The slightly oblique trajectory of the leg as it actively shifts backward serves to create a wider support base (i.e., a more solid, stable base). It activates the adductors to a greater degree than would happen with a parallel trajectory.

LORD BACKWARD LUNGE

Starting position

- **A |** Stand with legs together and arms at the sides.

Execution

- **B |** Compared to the previous exercise, you need to increase the rotation of the pelvis for this lunge. Rotate the hip and, following an inward diagonal trajectory, bring the right leg back well beyond the left leg's projection. You actually need to cross one leg behind the other with a medium-length step, creating an angle much greater than 180 degrees. The left foot rotates slightly. The end result should resemble the beginning of a curtsy.

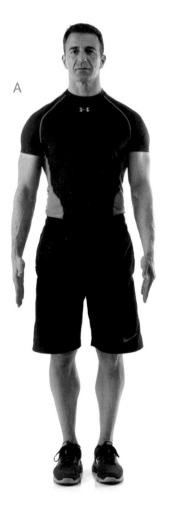

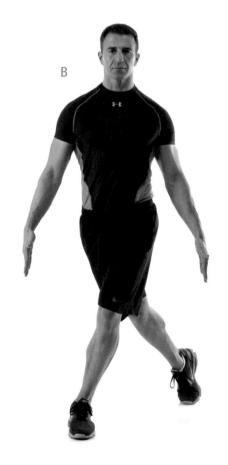

■ **C** | Bend the legs, lowering the right knee just behind the left heel (you will feel the left gluteus stretch).

■ **D** | Rise back up to the initial starting position and execute the exercise with the other leg.

Complete the required number of repetitions.

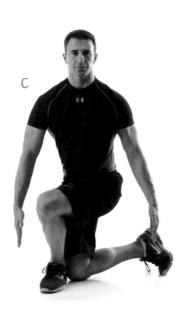

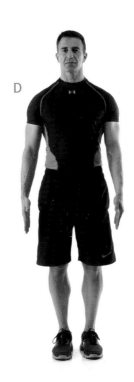

Discussion

The term *lord* is due to the fact that the movement imitates the curtsy used to pay homage to aristocrats. This movement requires great control during execution and, in the eccentric phase, greatly stretches the entire hip articulation and the muscles that insert also into the hip, including the knee and ankle. It is a great exercise for mobilization. It is valuable not only for those sports which put great stresses and loads on the joints, but also for combat, contact, and scrum sports such as wrestling, rugby, American football, and MMA. If carefully executed and included within an informal training program, it will be beneficial for all those who have strong dysmetria in the lower limbs or for athletes who are recovering from injuries and operations on the knee and hip. In the latter case, it should be included in the second part of any rehab program. A similar exercise preparatory to this is the in-line lunge, in which movement is forward and the feet advance on the same line. Balancing is easier but at the same time there is less stretching of the hip.

CROSS LUNGE

Starting position

- **A |** Stand with legs together, and take a step forward with the right leg.

Execution

- **B |** Lower the left knee until you brush the ground with it.

- **C and D |** Perform an upward jump,

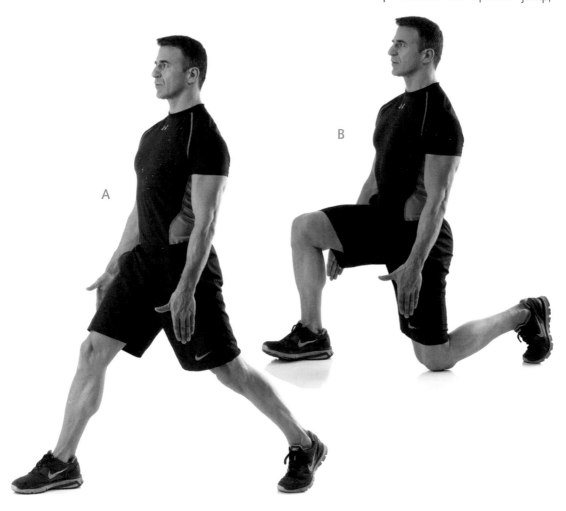

inverting the position of the legs (left leg forward, right leg backward) at the same time. Stabilize the position.

E | Repeat the exercise, this time lowering the right knee to the ground. Complete the required number of repetitions.

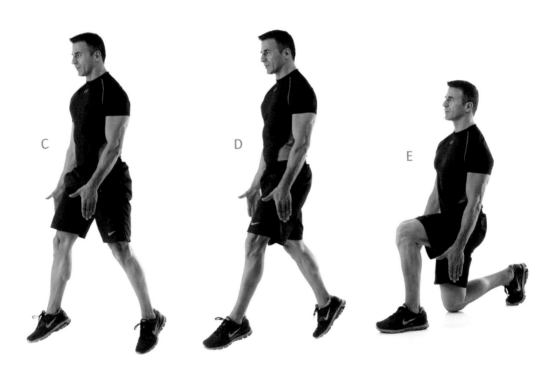

Discussion

Surely this exercise is to be included only after several months of athletic work. It fully satisfies the action and function of the hip extensor chain; besides, there is plyometric work involved (jumping and cushioning) and therefore great stress on the nerve components (fiber recruitment 2x). Add balance, motor coordination, and proprioception, and the picture is complete. A warning: All plyometric exercises have a decidedly strong impact on the muscle and tendon components, especially the tendons. For this reason, I believe it is important to limit the number of repetitions per set in this exercise to a maximum of 5. Of course, athletic training for performance sports may take you beyond this number, as you seek for those few but indispensable extra benefits you need to improve performance significantly. It is therefore important to remember that, as the list of benefits lengthens, so too does the list of risks. An athlete is aware of this, but a normal person isn't. Altogether, this is a good exercise to incorporate into a training program.

FROGGY JUMP

Starting position

- **A |** Squat down, crouching like a frog. The fingers touch the ground, and the back is straight and in the neutral position (do not bend forward).

Execution

- **B |** Jump upward, imitating a frog's movement. Control the return to the ground with a brief pause in the upright position for stabilization.

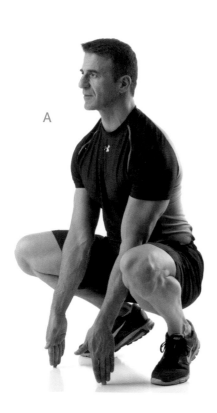

A

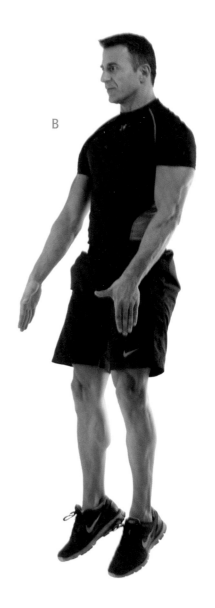

B

- **C and D |** Return to the squat position, then jump upward again. Complete the required number of repetitions.

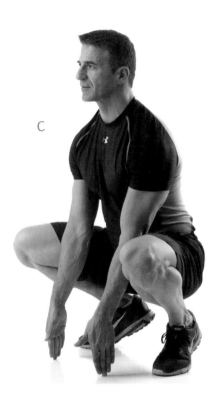

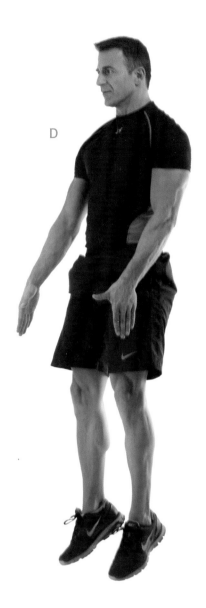

Discussion

As mentioned, plyometric exercises share a series of features which make them unique. Here we do have functionality: flexion and extension of the thigh and propulsion, action, and function of the hip extensor chain. Besides, this exercise works on the nerve components and therefore on recruitment. Simply: It works on strength! Proprioception, motor coordination, and spatial-temporal switching complete the picture. This is an underestimated exercise you should start using.

BURPEES

Starting position

- **A |** Squat down, crouching like a frog. The fingers touch the ground and the back is straight and in the neutral position (do not bend forward).

Execution

- **B |** While resting on the hands, extend the legs and the pelvis backward, with a little skip.

- **C |** Using elastic force, return to the initial position with another skip.

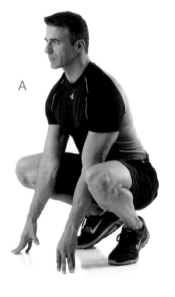
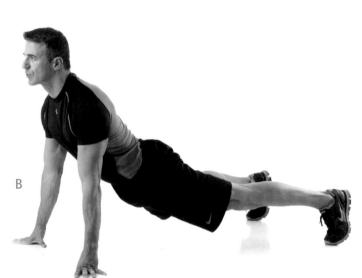

Discussion

Despite the name, Americans love burpees. It is a truly comprehensive exercise, a movement that is both dynamic and functional; it is functional because it combines action and function of the hip extensor chain. It is plyometric because the command signal reaches the muscle in a very short window of ca. 100 ms (Paillard[2], 1982). Burpees require a really significant cardiovascular and cardiorespiratory effort, too. In the US, this exercise is used as a test to measure the endurance strength of an athlete. The interesting feature of ballistic exercises (which include plyometrics) for athletes and sportspeople in all disciplines, from bodybuilding to running, lies in the fact that they seem to subvert Henneman's[3] law.

2 Paillard J. (1982). Apraxia and the neurophysiology of motor control, in *Philosophical Transactions of the Royal Society B: Biological Sciences*, 298: pp. 111-134

3 Henneman E., Somjen G., and Carpenter DO. (1965). Functional significance of cell size in spinal motoneurons, in *Journal of Neurophysiology*, 28: 560-580.

- **D |** Now jump upward, clapping the hands above your head. Land and stabilize your position. Squat once more and start all over again.

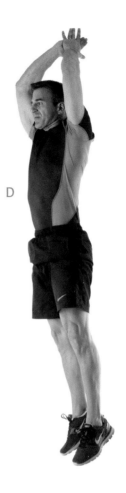

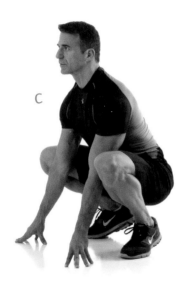

In short, Henneman's[4] law (1965) says that when you lift a load during an exercise, the first fibers to be activated are the red, type I fibers; as fatigue sets in, intermediate IIa fibers (fast oxidative glycolytic fibers) join in, and finally, when we reach our limit, IIx (fast-twitch) fibers join in. According to studies on high-jumpers and subsequently on other categories of athletes, it was demonstrated that ballistic exercise subverts this law. Faced with a body weight corresponding to more or less 40% of the maximum, strong electromyographic activity indicated the activation of type IIx fibers. So? So just do it, and include it in any training program: It works!

---

4 Henneman E. and Olson CB. (1965). Relations between structure and function in the design of skeletal muscles, in *Journal of Neurophysiology*, 28: 581-598. – Henneman E, Somjen G, and Carpenter DO. (1965). Excitability and inhibitability of motoneurons of different sizes, in *Journal of Neurophysiology*, 28: 599-620.

ONE-LEG KICK

Starting position

- **A |** Stand with your legs a little more than shoulder-width apart.
  Raise the right arm above your head.

Execution

- **B |** Squat down until you can place the right hand on the ground.

- **C |** Lower the pelvis a bit more and extend the right leg with a lateral trajectory between the right arm and the left leg.

- **D |** With one single movement, bring the right leg back to the initial squat position.

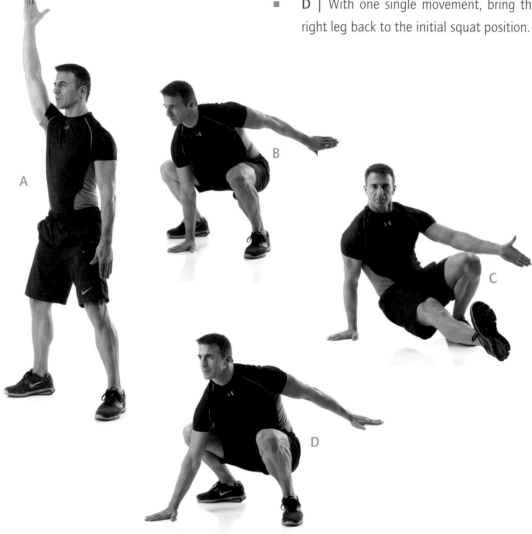

- **E |** Stand up, lifting the right hand off the ground and raising the left arm.

- **F |** Repeat the motion on the other side. The left arm goes down during the squat until the hand rests on the ground.

- **G |** Extend the left leg with a diagonal trajectory between the left arm and the right leg.

- **H |** With one single movement bring the left leg back to the squat position. Stand up again, raising the right hand high, and start again until you complete the required number of repetitions.

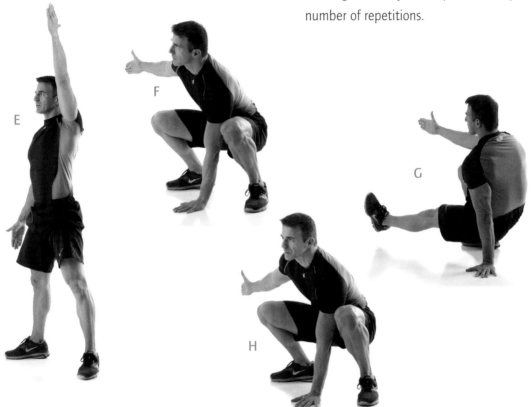

Discussion

This exercise is very compelling both in terms of coordination and proprioception. It is also cardiovascular, given the chains it involves. It features action and function of both the coxofemoral and its synergistic joints. I regard it as a mobilization exercise. In other words, it is suitable for unblocking and regaining flexibility in articular systems which are often little used, or at least little functionally. The complexity of the movement and of the muscular chains involved is confirmed by the work to which the cardiovascular and cardiorespiratory systems are subjected.

JUMPING JACK

Starting position

- A | Stand with your arms at the sides.

Execution

- B | Jump out and in by opening and closing the legs.

  At the same time, abduct the arms laterally and upward.

  Complete the required number of repetitions.

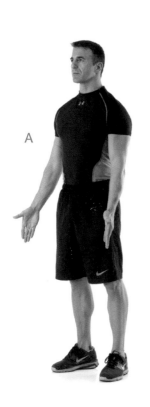
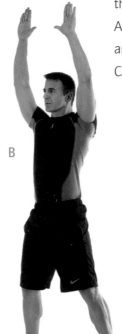

Discussion

This is widely used as a warm-up exercise, but don't underestimate the jumping jack. First of all, it is a plyometric exercise, requiring coordination and motor control besides significantly working by the cardiocirculatory and cardiovascular systems. It is excellent when inserted between exercises in circuits, and it is also an integral part of training programs involving dynamic lower-body work. Besides this, it is very effective for the whole musculature of the calf and for the synergy it requires from the tarsal-metatarsal, sub-astragalus, and tibial-tarsal joints. To be clear, if this synergy doesn't exist, you may have developed all your muscular chains, but you will still have poor propulsion. Think about this sequence:

1. Fast jumping jack 1 x 20 sec. 2. High jump 1 x 20 sec. 3. Skip 1 x 20 sec. 4. Burpees 1 x 20 sec. 5. Repeat the sequence 3-5 times. Trying is believing!

SEAL JACK

Starting position

- A | Stand with your legs together and extend the arms in front of you.

Execution

- B | Jump in and out by opening and closing the legs. At the same time, clap your hands in front of you.

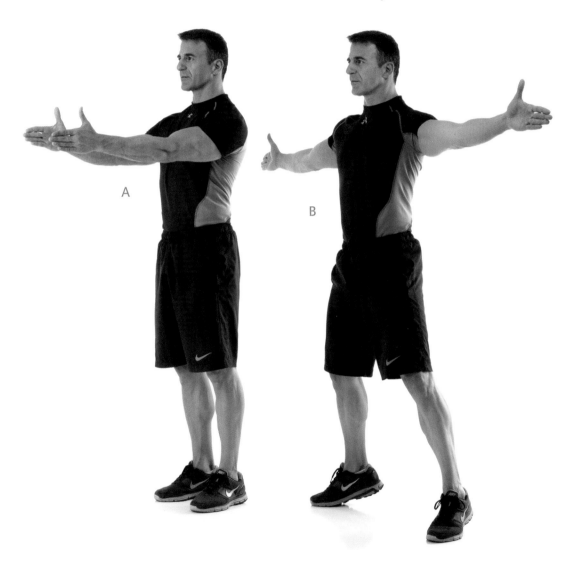

The same that was said for the jumping jack holds true for the seal jack. This exercise's evolution involves crossing the legs in the leg-closing phase, bringing them alternately forward. As the exercise evolves, so, too, does its difficulty.

GATE JACK

Starting position

- **A** | Stand with the arms at the sides.

Execution

- **B** | Even though the movement is apparently similar to the jumping jacks, it isn't exactly the same. Here you don't jump upward, opening your legs, but you let yourself fall down, opening the legs; at the same time, you grip your knees with your hands; then you stop at the bottom; and then you jump to close the legs and return to the starting position.

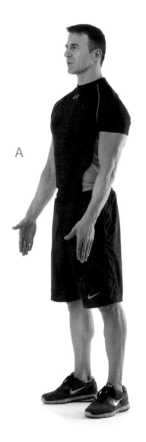

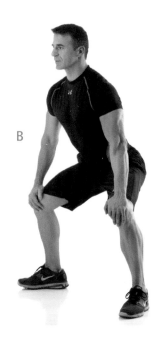

Discussion

What is interesting about this exercise is that it reverses a sequence—dynamic muscles, decelerator muscles—that is normally employed in sports performances. This is something you feel in your nervous system. Turning our attention to the eccentric phase of the exercise, another interesting feature is that more tension is developed upon the muscular chains involved; you will notice it in just a few jumps. This is another underestimated exercise that needs to be rediscovered.

SKIP

Starting position

- **A** | Stand with your legs together and the arms at the sides.

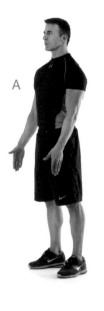

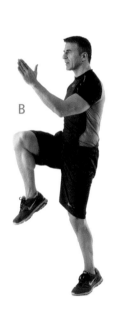

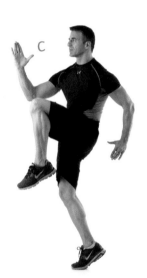

Execution

Skipping is almost like running in place. Almost.

- **B** | Start running in place, raising your knees as high as possible.

- **C** | Follow the movement of the lower limbs synergistically and alternately with your arms: right leg us, left arm up; left leg up, right arm up.

Discussion

Skipping is a time exercise with great cardiovascular and cardiorespiratory involvement. Its intensity is managed by the actual frequency of the steps run in place. If you try to accelerate running in place as much as possible, you will feel the effectiveness of this exercise. Not surprisingly, skipping is included in all pre-athleticism and athletic training protocols. Alternating low and high frequency is excellent for fully engaging all organic systems. Personally, I also use the skip to test a person's sporting history. Let me explain. Running is a gesture that belongs to us from infancy, or so it should. Yet, however simple the movement may seem, ask a sedentary person or someone who has started practicing sports after the age of 14 to do it. He or she will look clumsy, awkward, and uncoordinated. This tells a lot about his or her past and about the approach to use with this type of person. Hats off to this exercise.

STARTER

Starting position

- **A |** Set up in the sprinter crouching position, with hands resting on the ground in front of you and legs behind you, one slightly ahead of the other.

Execution

- **B and C |** While remaining with the hands on the ground, extend the lower limbs alternately, mimicking a run. Execute for the length of time required.

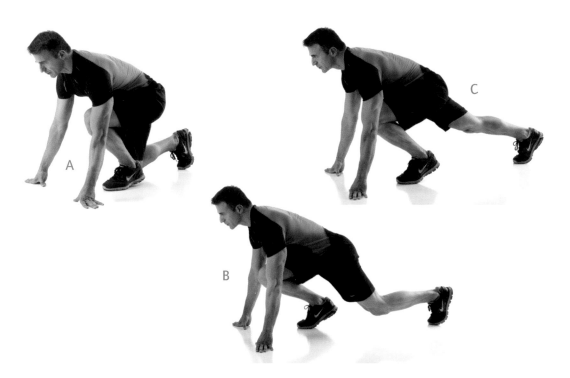

This exercise involves a high cardiovascular effort, and at the same time it works on the core and the scapula stabilizers. It is a good exercise suitable for inclusion in circuit training for rugby, American football, wrestling, MMA, combat sports, and tennis. A mini-circuit I have used for tennis players in the final part of their training is the following:

1. Skip 20 sec
2. Starter 20 sec
3. Jumping jack 20 sec
4. Gate jack 20 sec
5. Repeat the sequence 5-10 times.

KNEELING JUMP

Starting position A

- Kneel on the ground, the glutes away from the heels and the arms at your sides.

Execution

- With an explosive movement of the hips, helped by the arms, gather momentum and jump to your feet, finding yourself in a full squat.
Return to the starting position.
Complete the required number of repetitions.

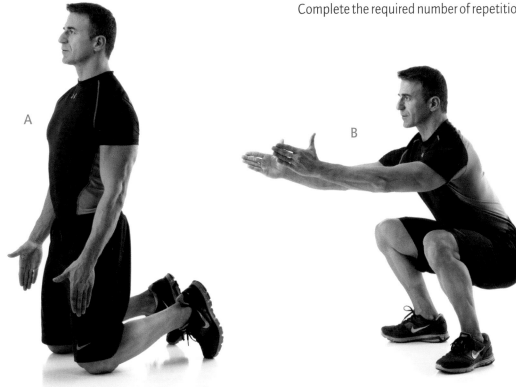

Discussion

The kneeling jump is a fantastic exercise to reinforce the action and function of the coxofemoral joint and the kinematic chains connected to it. I was taught this exercise by the great coach Martin Rooney. Any sport featuring power, explosiveness, and other expressions of speed strength will find the movement in this exercise highly advantageous for training. It may also be executed in combination with a barbell deadlift or a kettlebell snatch. Circle it in red!

KNEELING DOUBLE JUMP

Starting point

- A | Kneel on the ground, the glutes away from the heels and the arms at your sides.

Execution

- B | With an explosive movement of the hips, helped by the arms, gather momentum and jump to your feet, landing almost in a full squat.

- C | From this position, gather new momentum and jump as high as possible. Land and return to the kneeling position. Repeat performing the required number of repetitions.

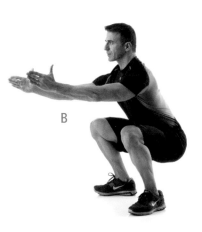

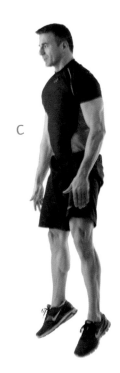

Discussion

This fantastic exercise involves a double plyometric movement, which is exceptional for working on explosive force. The kneeling double jump is well suited for sports such as basketball, volleyball, beach volleyball, rugby, American football, powerlifting, martial and combat arts, MMA. It works not only on the nerve components but also on the muscular components. The fact that it consequentially trains other motor qualities and skills is not to be underestimated. It may also be executed in combination with a barbell deadlift or a kettlebell snatch.

HALF-KNEELING CROSS JUMP

Starting position

- **A |** Set up in a half-kneeling position, with the right knee and the left foot resting on the ground and arms at the sides.

Execution

- **B and C |** Gathering momentum, helped by the arms, jump upward, inverting the position of the legs.

- **D |** Return to the starting position, slowing down your descent to avoid hitting the knee on the ground. Complete the required number of repetitions.

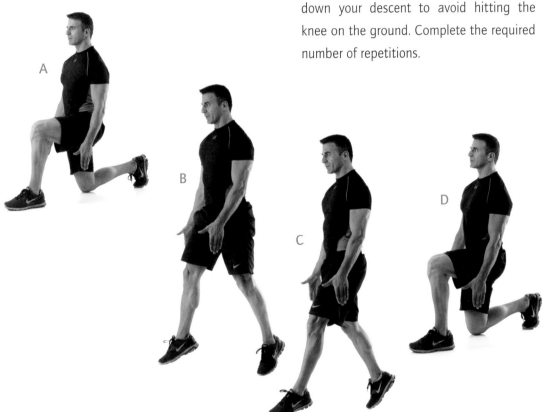

Discussion

This exercise works explosive strength some more, with the addition of a highly-controlled eccentric movement phase. This is a functional exercise. What was mentioned for the kneeling double jump holds true with this exercise, with an important difference: Balance and proprioception on the sagittal plane are stimulated to a greater degree, and the training stimulus is greater, at least if we execute the exercise with body weight. I believe that two annual plyometric exercise mesocycles ought always to be included in the athletic training for intermediate and advanced athletes.

ALTERNATING HALF-LUNGE

Starting position

- A | Set up in a half-kneeling position, with the left knee and the right foot resting on the ground and your arms extended forward.

Execution

- B | Raise the legs slightly, lifting the left knee off the ground. Lean the torso forward; this self-contained position must be held throughout the exercise.

- C | Now start inverting the position of the legs, slowly at first then faster, keeping the body and the center of gravity low. The torso keeps leaning slightly forward.

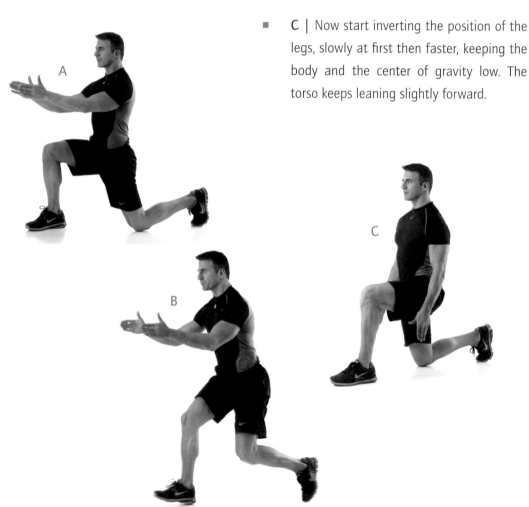

Discussion

In many sports, the functionality of the hip extensor chain is limited by its weakest link, the quadriceps. This exercise stimulates the quadriceps in a tough, functional way and strengthens them progressively.

10.5   CORE TRAINING

ROPE CRUNCH

Starting position

- **A |** Lie supine on the ground, knees bent and forming a 90-degree angle. Place a rope beneath the lower back and rest your hands, closed in a fist, behind the nape.

Execution

- **B |** Exhaling, lift the upper torso and shoulders with a controlled movement, bringing the ribs and the pelvis closer.
  Inhaling, slowly bring the torso and shoulders back down to the ground.
  Complete the required number of repetitions.

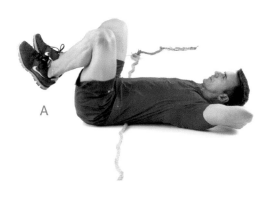

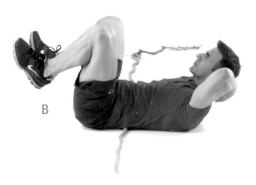

Discussion

Americans have branded the classic crunch exercise performed in gyms as foolish and dangerous. Reluctantly, I cannot fault them. The most authoritative biomechanics and anatomy texts say that a semi-rigid structure like the spine, formed by several mobile segments next to each other, can bear more tension the more curves it features on its course. Now, with the classic crunch in the imprint position (i.e., with the spine lying flat on the ground), we lose at least one of these curves: the lumbar hinge. We are therefore more vulnerable precisely in that segment where there is the greatest stress from the forces acting from below (during walking) and from above (the weight of the trunk and the upper body). Using a rope beneath the lumbar spine will keep the spine in a neutral position, preserving its integrity. You will notice that, curiously, the rope will not bother or hurt, and that, on the contrary, the exercise's difficulty will be greatly increased.

ROPE V-CRUNCH

Starting position

- **A** | Lie supine on the ground, the knees raised and bent at a 45-degree angle. Place a rope beneath the lumbar spine.
  Extend the arms upward and bring the chin close to your chest (about 4 in. [10 cm]

- **B** | Exhaling, lift up with both arms and torso toward an imaginary point to the side of the right foot, with slow, controlled movement. Descend slowly, inhaling.

- **C** | Exhaling, lift up with the arms and torso toward an imaginary point to the side of the left foot. Descend slowly, inhaling, and repeat, completing the required number of repetitions.

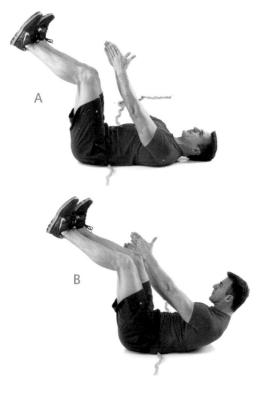

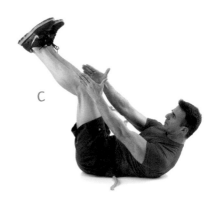

Discussion

What was said for the previous exercise regarding the spine's neutral position and the rope's help still holds true. Another peculiarity is the trajectory the body must follow during the exercise: It is a tight V, with no special rotations, and it follows the oblique muscles' innervations and allows them to contract more. The origin and the insertion draw much closer compared with other executions. You will immediately feel the result: a full stimulus to the abdominal fascia, including the "low abdominals! I hope I will not hear this term any more...

REVERSE ROPE CRUNCH

Starting position

- **A |** Lie supine on the ground, the knees pulled into the chest. Place a rope beneath the lumbar spine and place your fists behind the head.

Execution

- **B |** Exhaling, flex the pelvis and bring it upward, closer to the thorax, with a slow, controlled movement.
  Inhaling, return slowly to the ground.
  Complete the required number of repetitions.

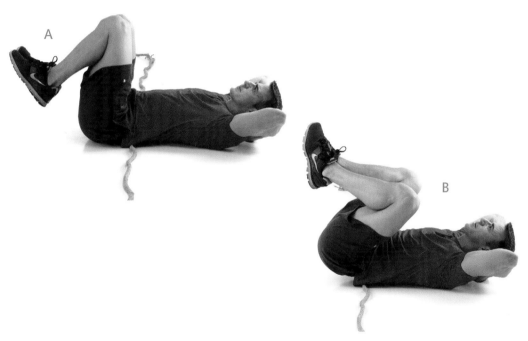

Discussion

This is a difficult exercise, which requires a well-trained, efficient, and strong abdominal fascia. Point one: The hands are behind the head and not anchored to some wall bar or the ground, so you don't have the chance to use the arms or trapezius to help complete the exercise. Point two: In order to be more effective, the movement needs to be coordinated with breathing. Point three: The load rests almost fully on the rectus abdominis, involving the sub-umbilical and supra-umbilical fibers sequentially. Point four: The rope contributes to making the exercise harder. This is one of the exercises used to test the real strength of the rectus abdominis. I have met several coaches who had great difficulty in performing it and who have adopted it for this reason.

PLANK

Starting position and execution

- **A** | Lie prone on the ground. Rest the forearms on the ground with the elbows perpendicular below the shoulders; the feet are at 90-degree angles to the legs.
  Imagine your body is a plank and raise it, lining up the legs, pelvis, and trunk. The support points are the forearms and the tips of your feet.

Slightly contract the abdomen, closing in the ribs and bringing them toward the pelvis.
Stay in position for the preset time.

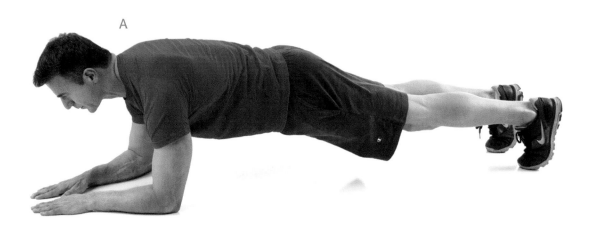

Discussion

In gyms, abdominal fascia training has become a soap opera: "1001 Ways of Doing Crunches". On the contrary, the abdominal fascia's first function is trunk stabilization, followed by lateral flexion, rotation, and respiration. This is the simplest and most straightforward exercise to train it. It is important that the elbows are perpendicular to the shoulders and the back is in the neutral position (i.e., the physiological curves are maintained). Here the rectus abdominis is one of the main stabilizing muscles and the first antagonist of the quadratus lumborum. If yours gives way, you will immediately feel stress and tension in the lower back. This is a great, often underestimated, exercise. Perhaps because it is too simple?

SIDE PLANK

Starting position

- **A |** In a lateral recumbent position, set the right forearm on the ground, with the shoulder perpendicular to the elbow; the feet are overlapping.
  Raise the left arm, pointing it straight upward.

Execution

- **B |** Imagine you are a plank and lift the pelvis upward. You will be resting on the outside of the right foot and on the right forearm.
  Stay in position for the tension time required, at least 10 sec.
  Repeat on the other side, leaning on the left forearm.

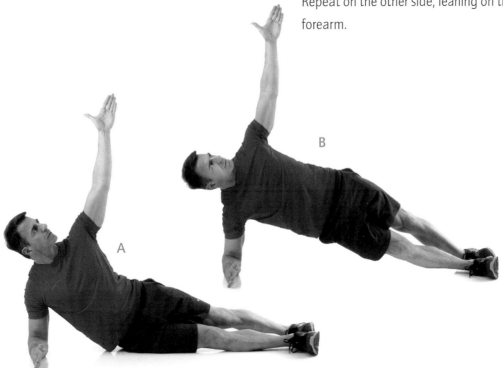

Discussion

This is an evolution of the previous exercise. It requires comparatively more control and stimulates the oblique muscles on either side more than the plank. It also strengthens the humerus and scapula stabilizers, the rotator cuff, and the paravertebral muscles. This is another movement, which, mysteriously, is little used and highly underestimated though it allows fast progress. Aesthetically, the effects on the waistline are significant and visible in a short time.

ALL FOUR AND TWIST

Starting position

- **A |** In a quadrupedal position, bend the left arm and bring the left hand behind the neck.

Execution

- **B |** With a slight contraction of the abdomen, rotate the left torso and arm medially inward, bringing the left elbow slightly behind the right elbow.

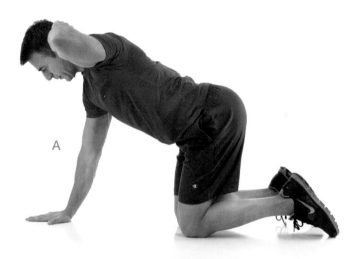

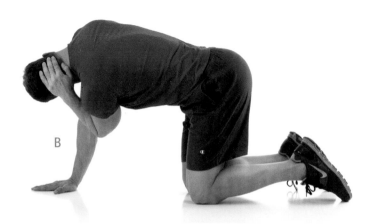

- **C |** Return slowly to the starting position, but don't stop. Continue the rotation until the tension will stop you.

- **D and E |** Repeat for the required number of repetitions, and complete the exercise by performing the rotation on the opposite side.

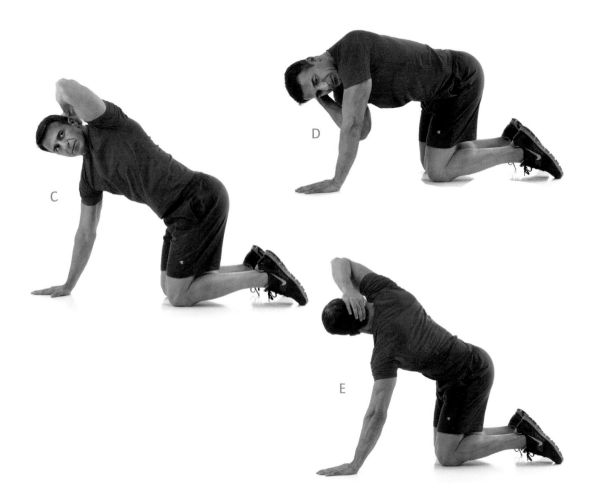

Discussion

Brett Klika, a clever young Californian coach, taught me this exercise. It looks easy, but it isn't. The crucial issue is the contraction of the rectus abdominis, the real antagonist of the quadratus lumborum. Here it ensures that the execution is correct and the back is protected. Keep it contracted, and it will automatically limit torso rotation (contraindicated otherwise) and train the abdominal fascia; loosen it, and the back will soon suffer for it. Trying is believing!

PLANK TWIST

Starting position

- **A** | Lie down in the prone position, the forearms on the ground and the elbows perpendicular below the shoulders; the feet are at 90-degree angles to the legs.
  Imagine your body is a plank and lift it, lining up the legs, pelvis, and trunk; the support points are the forearms and the tips of your feet.

Execution

- **B** | Now, supporting yourself forward on the right forearm, bend the left arm and bring the left hand behind the neck.

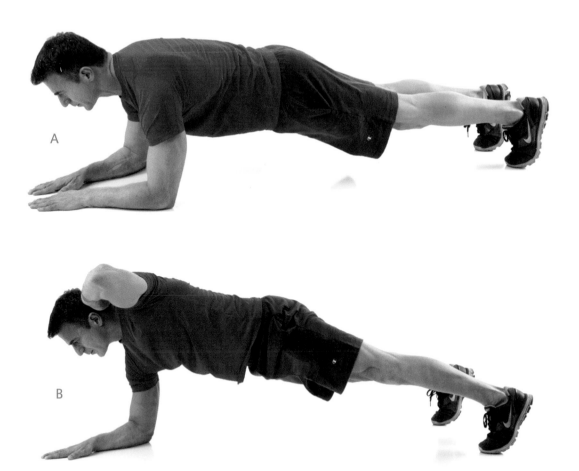

■ **C |** Keeping a three-point support—both feet and the right forearm—rotate the torso slightly and touch the right elbow with the left elbow (without letting it touching the ground).

■ **D |** Return to the starting position and complete the required number of repetitions. Then perform it on the other side, bending the right arm and supporting yourself on the left forearm.

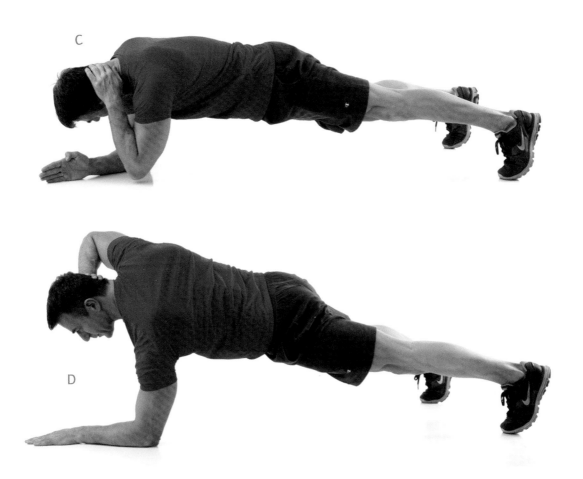

Discussion

This is a highly engaging exercise not suitable for beginners. Stabilization, rotation, and flexion: The exercise has it all. It is one of the best exercises for strengthening the abdominal fascia. The key issue is keeping the pelvis stable in position despite two destabilizing factors: 1. only using three limbs as support; and 2. trunk rotation.

SIDE PLANK WITH TWIST

Starting position

- **A |** In a lateral recumbent position, place the right forearm on the ground, with the elbow perpendicular to the shoulder; the feet are overlapping.

  Lift the left arm and bend it, bringing the left hand behind the neck.

  Imagine you are a plank and lift the pelvis up. You will be supported by the outside of the right foot and the right forearm.

Execution

- **B |** Now, with a controlled movement, rotate the torso, bringing the left elbow toward the right elbow, without resting it on the ground.

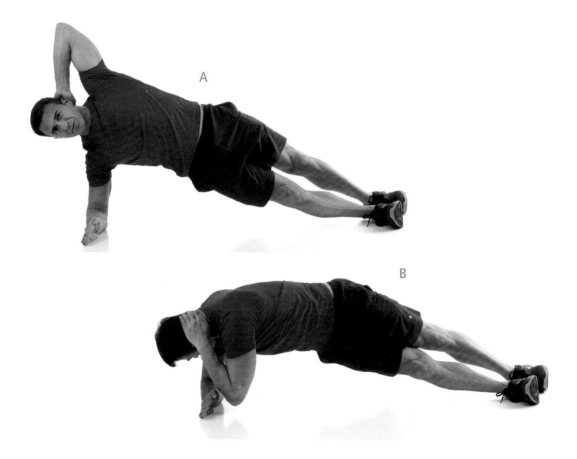

A

B

- **C |** Return to the starting position and complete the required number of repetitions. Repeat on the other side.

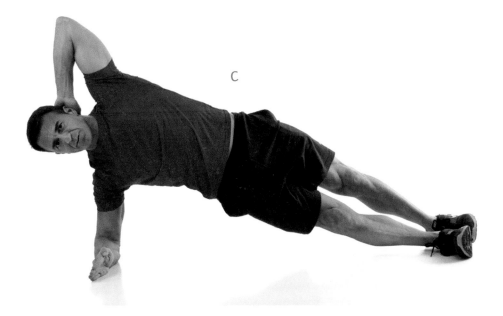

C

Discussion

This is a good functional exercise. The abdominal fascia is really challenged, especially the transversus and the internal and external oblique muscles. Also, balance and coordination are thoroughly trained. It is useful for preparing the body for heavy lifting and excellent for all those sports in which torso rotations and flexion are needed, such as rugby, American football, basketball, combat arts, martial arts, volleyball, beach volleyball, football, and even archery.

SIDE PLANK WITH ROTATION

Starting position

- **A |** In a lateral recumbent position, place the right forearm on the ground, with the elbow perpendicular to the shoulder; the feet overlap.
  Raise the left arm, pointing it straight upward.

Execution

- **B |** Imagine you are a plank and lift the pelvis up. You will be supported by the outside of the right foot and the forearm.

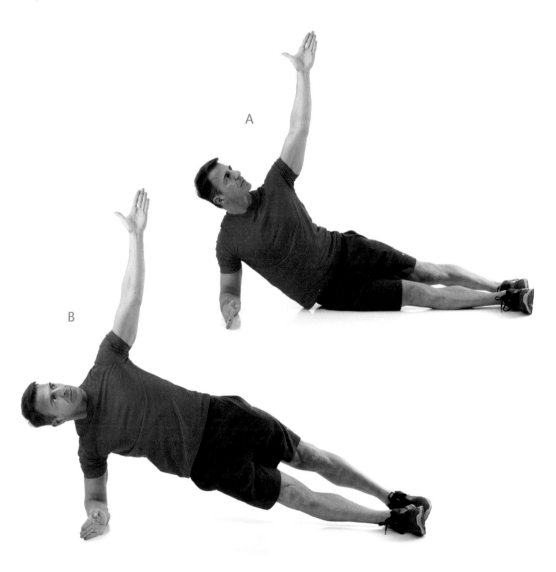

■ **C |** Rotate the torso slowly, moving the left arm toward the right, into the space between the torso and the floor. The feet remain stationary; the rotation depends wholly on the hips and the pelvis. Turn back up slowly, complete the repetitions required, and repeat on the other side.

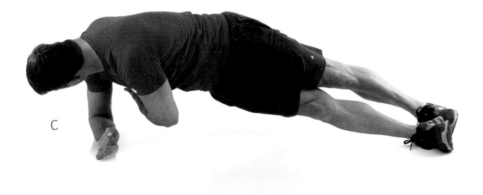

C

Discussion

This is probably the best exercise for the transversus and oblique muscles. It features stabilization, rotation and flexion of the abdominal fascia, as well as a very hefty stimulus to the scapula stabilizers and the rotator cuff muscles. Because the torso changes position during the exercise, the rotator cuffs are needed more for stabilization. In the same manner, the whole paravertebral musculature joins the action.

LEOPARD PLANK

Starting position

- **A |** Adopt the plank position; rest on your forearms and the tips of your feet, which will be at 90-degree angles to the legs. Close your hands in a fist and bring them close together.

Execution

- **B |** Keeping the pelvis low and in line, move both the left forearm and the right leg forward at the same time.

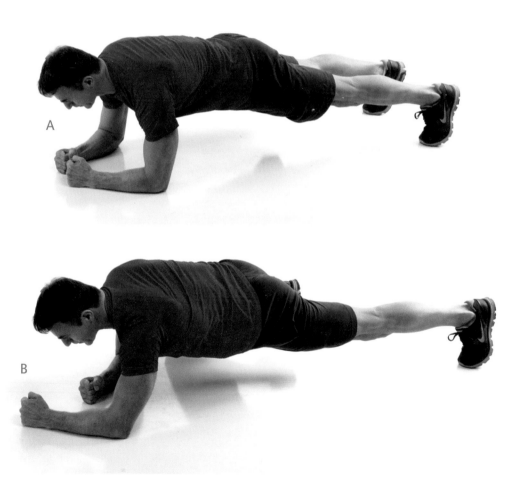

- **C** | Pivot on the left forearm and the right foot to bring the right arm and left leg forward.

- **D** | Continue the movement to cover the set distance.

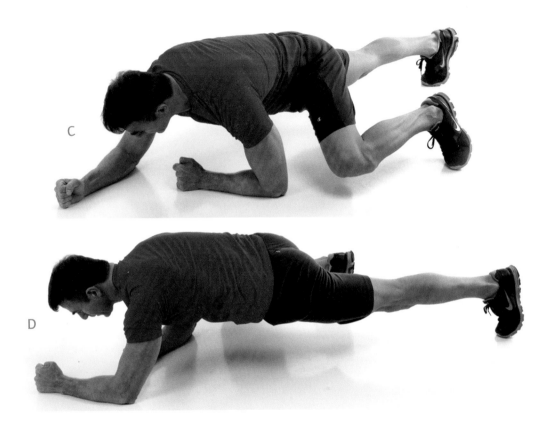

Discussion

This is a highly dynamic movement that involves the whole abdominal fascia. In terms of motor patterns, the leopard plank is reminiscent of the army crawl, with the minor difference that you don't rest for support on the whole of the lower and upper arms, but rather on the tip of the foot and the forearm only. The body is suspended, and the core muscles are constantly contracted. This is an excellent functional exercise because it involves stabilization, flexion, and rotation, as well as coordination, proprioception, and balance. Also, this is a fun exercise, suitable for different training objectives. Don't underestimate this exercise, either. I use it as a transition in core circuits. For example, I choose a crunch exercise and another one for stationary stabilization, and I use the leopard plank as an interlude between them. Circle it in red.

SIDEWALK PLANK

Starting position

- **A |** Assume the plank position; rest on your forearms and the tips of your feet, which will be at 90-degree angles to the legs. Close your hands in a fist and bring them close together.

Execution

- **B |** Maintaining the starting position, slowly shift the body laterally, following this sequence: right leg—

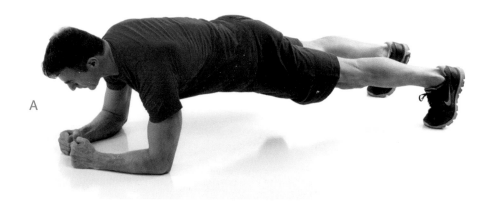

A

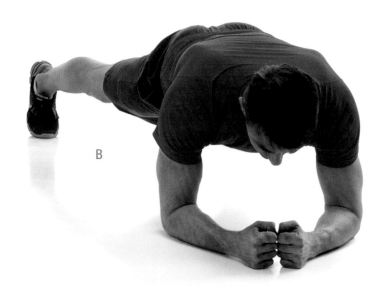

B

- **C |** —right arm—

- **D |** —left arm—left leg. Perform 5-10 shifts in one direction, then double back.

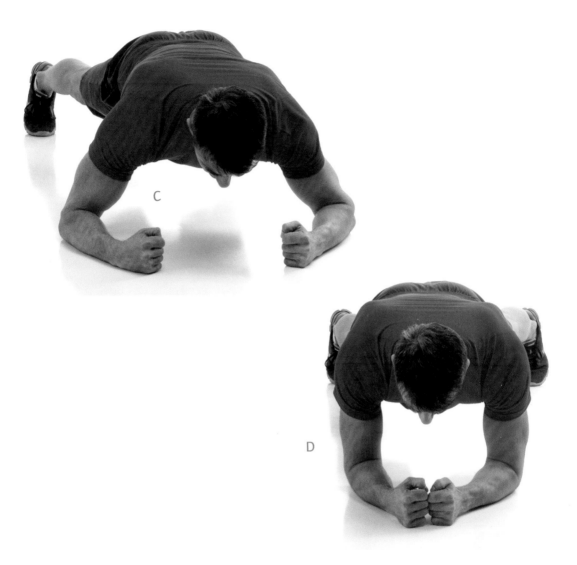

Discussion

This exercise doesn't require a complex gesture, but it is highly intense, because of the control and tension it imparts on the kinematic chains involved. Shifting the body while maintaining tension in the abdominal fascia isn't easy; besides, shifting involves all the core muscles. Once again, the stabilization of the rectus abdominis is crucial for a correct execution, since it protects the lumbar hinge. Needless to say: This is an excellent exercise.

CRAB PLANK

Starting position

- **A |** Adopt the plank position, with arms straight.

Execution

- **B and C |** Holding the starting position, slowly shift your body laterally following this sequence: right leg—left arm—

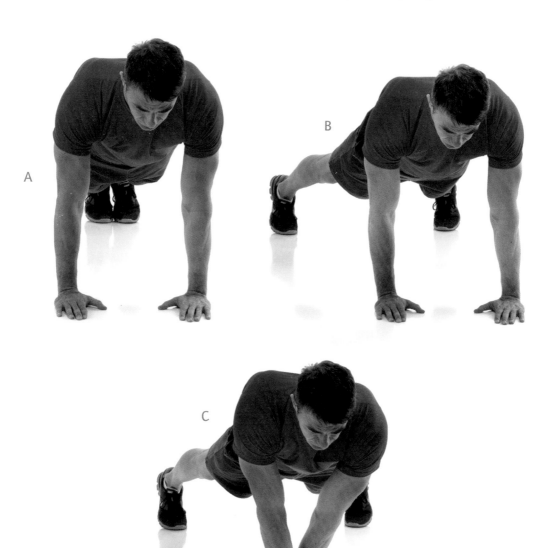

- **D and E** | —right arm—left leg. Perform 5-10 shifts in one direction, and then double back.

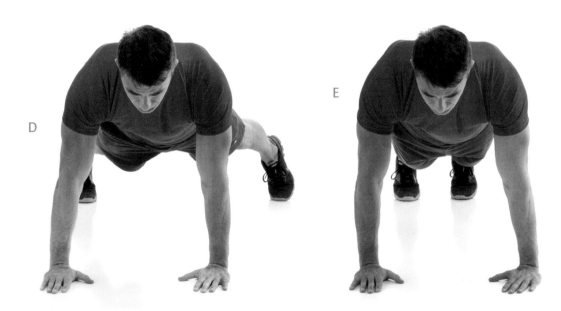

Discussion

What was said for the previous exercise holds true, with the difference being that you are supporting your body on your hands and not the forearms. In biomechanical terms, straight arms imply the involvement of two extra joints compared to the previous exercise: the elbow and wrist joints. This means there are four extra systems involved in applying tension to the ground (the joints and articular capsules). In summary: The triceps is involved by the extension of the forearm, and the pectoralis and latissimus dorsi contribute to trunk stabilization. The pectoralis also works every time the arms cross over, performing its typical action: flexion on the transverse plane.

PLANK WITH SIDE-LEG FLEX

Starting position

■ **A** | Adopt the plank position, the hands close to each other and resting on the ground on their side.

Execution

■ **B** | Holding the initial position, flex the right thigh laterally, trying to bring it closer to the right arm.

■ **C** | Return to the starting position and repeat with the other leg. Complete the required number of repetitions (at least 5 on each side).

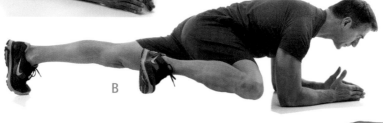

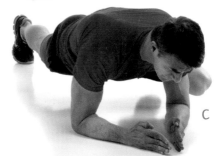

Discussion

This is an excellent core exercise, specifically for the oblique muscles, which are highly stimulated here. Concentrate on the trunk and pelvis position. Close the ribs slightly, bringing them nearer the pelvis and contracting the rectus abdominis. This is your basic position; the lateral movement of the legs must not distract you from this objective. It is a basic movement which is very effective in athletic training for all, I repeat all, sports, but also for general health and well-being. Circle it in red.

PLANK ON ARMS WITH FRONT-LEG FLEX

Starting position

- A | Adopt the plank position, with arms straight.

Execution

- B | Holding the basic position, flex the right thigh forward, bringing the knee toward the chest.

- C | Return to the starting position.

- D | Perform the same movement with the left leg.

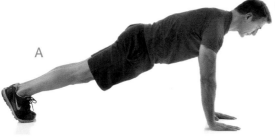

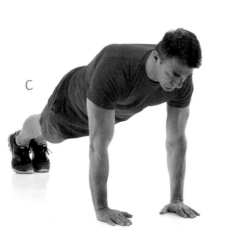

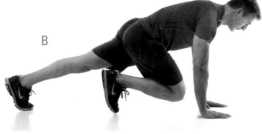

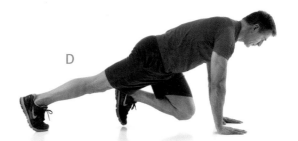

Discussion

What was said for the previous exercise holds true. The straight-arms position allows for a greater release of tension from the spine. The entire core demands stabilization, so you add the dynamic contraction of the rectus abdominis and the oblique muscles, which must fight the destabilization cause by the lower-body movement. This is undoubtedly an excellent exercise.

ARM-WALKING PLANK

Starting position

- **A |** Adopt the plank position with arms straight.
  Contract the rectus abdominis, closing the ribs in slightly toward the pelvis and pushing the navel (not the lumbar area) up

- **B |** Keeping the feet still, start advancing slowly, first with one arm—

- **C |** —and then with the other.

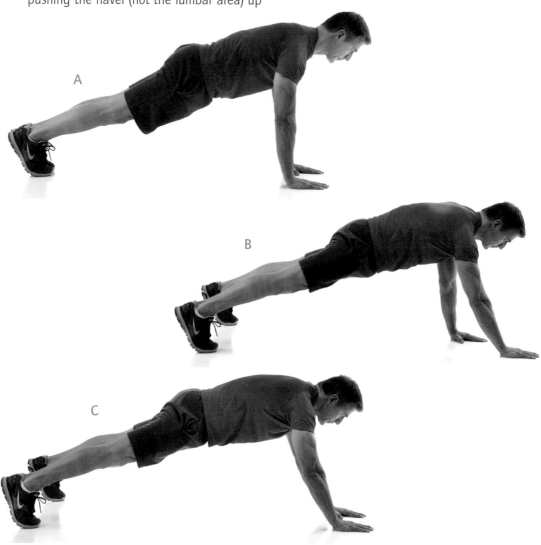

A

B

C

■ **D** | Keep advancing. You will feel a progressive increase in core activation.

■ **E** | Stop when tension is high. Hold the isometric contraction for 3 seconds then get back slowly.

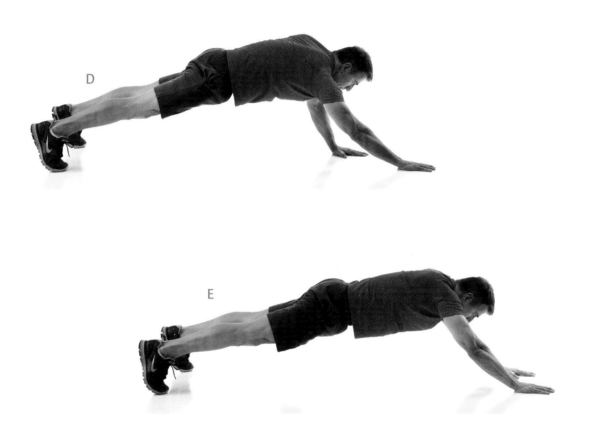

Discussion

This is one of the few exercises that tests the strength of the abdominal fascia. The intervention of the rectus abdominis as antagonist of the quadratus lumborum is essential. The whole load will rest on the lumbar hinge if the rectus abdominis isn't activated. Work by progressively increasing the stationary duration of the critical phase of the exercise.

STANDING KILLER CRUNCH

Starting position

- **A |** Stand with the legs farther apart than shoulder width.
  Extend the arms in front of the body at chest height, and interlock the hands, pointing the index and middle fingers.

Execution

- **B |** Contract the rectus abdominis, closing the ribs in slightly toward the pelvis, and quickly rotate arms and torso to the right.

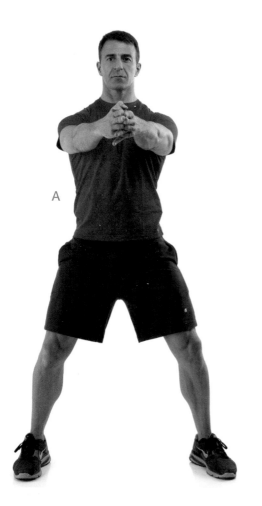

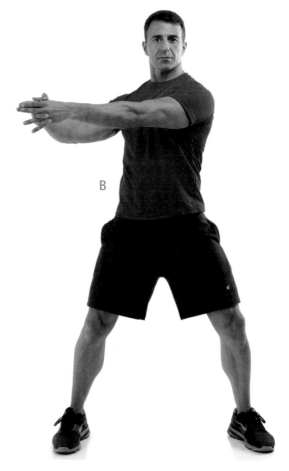

■ C | Complete the required number of repetitions (at least 5) and repeat on the opposite side.

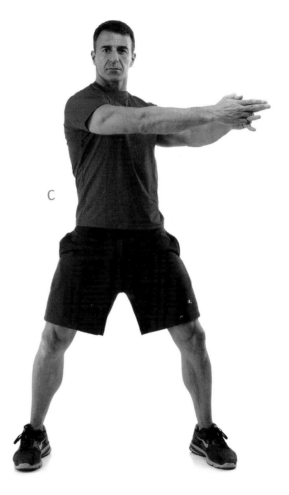

C

Discussion

We are bipeds. We must take the upright posture into account. We must accept this physiological reality and train our muscles standing up. In this exercise, the action of the rectus abdominis is essential to stabilize the trunk and protect the lumbar hinge. The activation of the transversus and oblique muscles is equally important, because they are dynamically involved in the exercise. When executing the movement, you must do more than a simple twist (a rotation from one side to the other). This type of exercise activates a nerve reflex, the myotatic reflex, which facilies the action of the muscles involved, eventually reducing their workload. Your objective is instead to rotate the trunk in one direction, return to the starting position, and then repeat the rotation on the same side again. Complete the number of required repetitions before performing an equal number of them on the opposite side.

STANDING BOXER CRUNCH

Starting position

- **A |** Stand with the legs at shoulder width and slightly flexed. Inhale and expand the abdomen.

Execution

- **B |** Exhale, compressing the abdomen in a decisive, powerful fashion, as though you are being punched in the stomach.
Repeat 3-5 times.

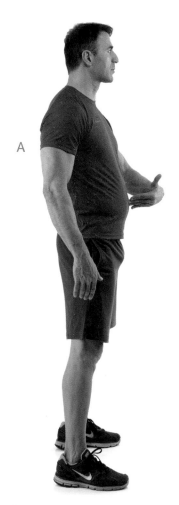
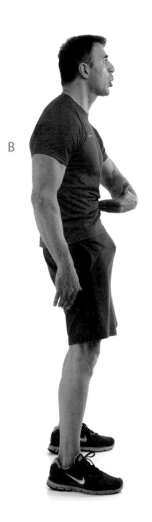

Discussion

The transversus muscle bears almost the entire workload. This exercise also stimulates the diaphragm, our essential respiratory muscle, which can easily lead to hyperventilation, dizziness, and a fall in tension. This explains the limited number of repetitions.

STANDING PITCHER CRUNCH

Starting position

- **A |** Stand, supporting yourself on the left leg only; the right leg is raised and bent. Extend the left arm forward and raise the right one.

Execution

- **B |** Imagine you are holding a stone in your right hand, and you have to throw it. Wind up the arm backward, above your head, rotating the torso from left to right.

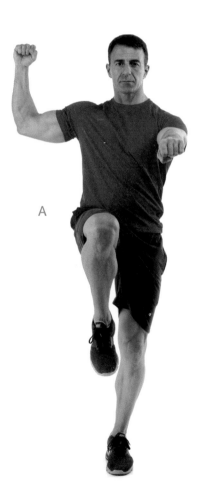

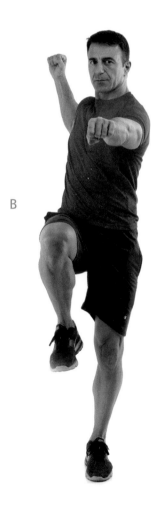

■ **C** | Keeping your balance, simulate throwing the imaginary stone fast and downward; the trajectory your hand will follow is a diagonal from above the head to the side of the left knee. Still taking care not to lose balance, raise the torso and complete the number of required repetitions (initially 3 to 5).

■ **D** | Return to the starting position, this time supported by the right leg, and get ready to perform the exercise on the opposite side.

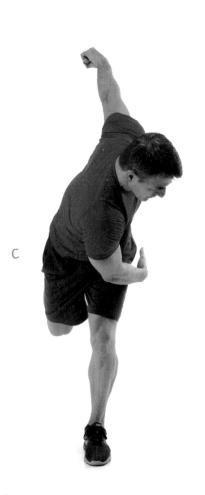

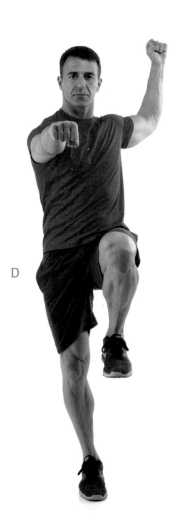

Discussion

There are few exercises as complex, complete, and engaging as this one. It isn't suitable for beginners, even though this motor gesture is widely used in a high number of sports and activities. This exercise has the entire works: proprioception, balance, coordination, stabilization, and engagement of the whole anterior cruciate chain and core. Let me underline the importance of the abdominal fascia both

■ **E |** Imagine you are holding a stone in your left hand and wind up the raised arm.

■ **F |** Throw the imaginary stone toward the low right-hand corner, taking care to maintain balance. Complete the required number of repetitions.

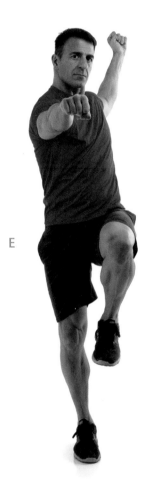

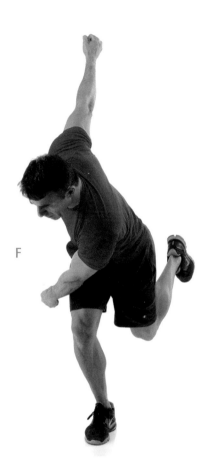

in the release and deceleration phase and when the movement is wound up again and the torso lifts up once more, extending upward. The action of the rectus abdominis is essential in this phase, since the body is destabilized. For this reason, you should flex the thigh that is the suspended toward the trunk when you rewind the movement by raising the torso; this movement will activate the rectus abdominis, allowing you to find stability and balance.

STANDING WOODCHOPPER CRUNCH

Starting position

- **A |** Stand with the legs at shoulder width, slightly flexed.

  Extend the arms to chest height in front of your body and interlock your hands, imagining you are wielding an ax.

  Inhaling, wind up the ax swing by stretching the arms in a diagonal trajectory toward the upper right-hand corner.

Execution

- **B |** Exhaling, contract the rectus abdominis and bring the arms toward the left side fast, following an oblique trajectory. Repeat 5 times.

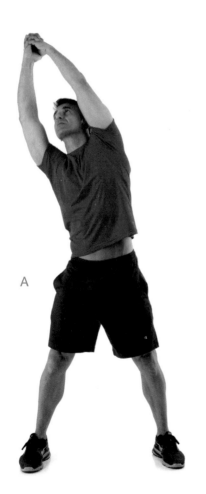

A

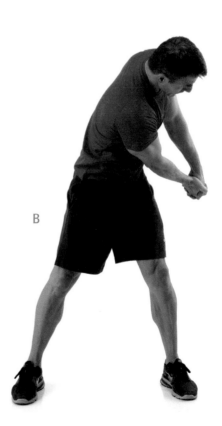

B

■ **C and D** | Execute another 5 times on the other side: Wind up by stretching toward the upper left-hand corner and release downward toward the opposite side.

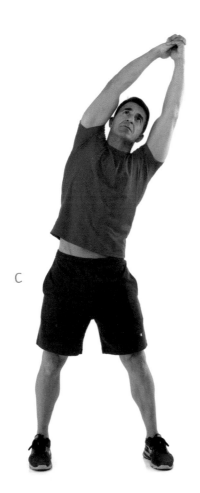
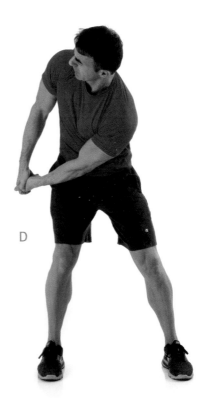

C

D

Discussion

The woodchopper crunch is a complete functional exercise in which the whole core is engaged. The rectus abdominis contributes to torso stabilization; the transversus is activated by the powerful inhalation; and the oblique muscles work diagonally throughout the fast contraction.

HALF-KNEELING MONSTER CRUNCH (WITH ELBOW OUT)

Starting position	Execution
■ **A** | Adopt a half-kneeling position: the right leg is bent and right foot resting on the ground, and the left leg is flexed, resting on the left knee and foot. Interlock your hands behind the neck.	■ **B** | Exhaling, flex the torso, bringing the left elbow across the body to the outside of the right knee.

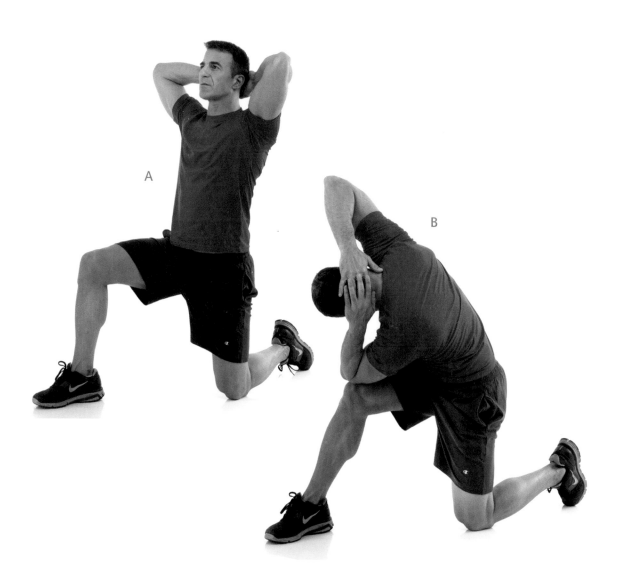

- **C** | Return to the starting position and repeat at least 10 times.

- **D** | Switch the legs' position and perform on the other side for the same number of repetitions.

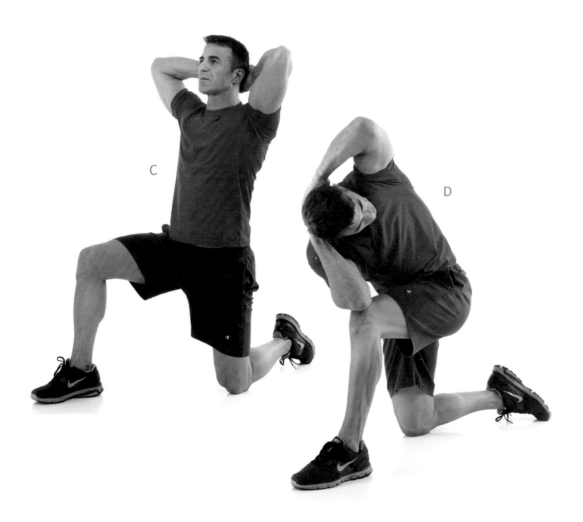

Discussion

This is a very simple exercise for starting the core's functional training. It is one of the first exercises to teach in order to activate the various components of the abdominal fascia, which come into play sequentially. It is also a fine mobilization exercise for the lumbar hinge and the pelvis.

HALF-KNEELING MONSTER CRUNCH (WITH ELBOW IN)

Starting position

- **A |** Adopt a half-kneeling position: the right leg is bent and the foot resting on the ground, and the left leg is flexed, resting on the knee and foot.
  Interlock your hands behind the neck.

Execution

- **B |** Exhaling, flex the torso, bringing the right elbow toward the inside of the right knee.

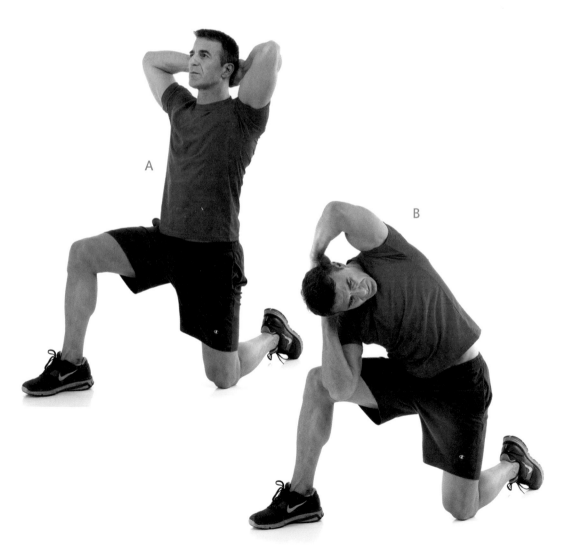

■ **C |** Return to the starting position and repeat at least 10 times.

■ **D |** Invert the legs' position and perform on the other side for the same number of repetitions.

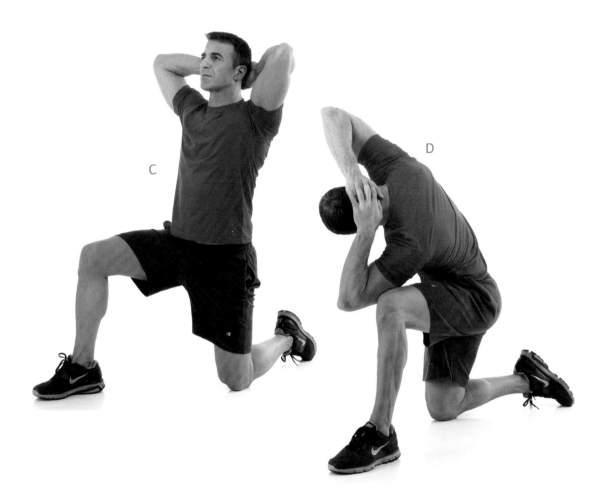

Discussion

The same that was said for the previous exercise holds true for this exercise. The main difference between in this exercise is in the stimulation of the oblique muscles. In the previous exercise, you work the large oblique muscle a little more. In this exercise you work the small oblique muscle more. The rest of the core is fully activated. Both variations are excellent for learning abdominal fascia activation. It is also a mobilization exercise for the lumbar hinge and the pelvis.

HALF-KNEELING KILLER CRUNCH

Starting position

- **A |** Adopt a half-kneeling position: the right leg is bent and the foot resting on the ground, and the left leg is flexed, the knee and foot resting on the ground.
  Extend the arms at chest height in front of your body and interlock the hands.

Execution

- **B |** Exhaling, contract the rectus abdominis to stabilize the torso; then rotate your arms and trunk fast to the right. Perform 5-10 times.

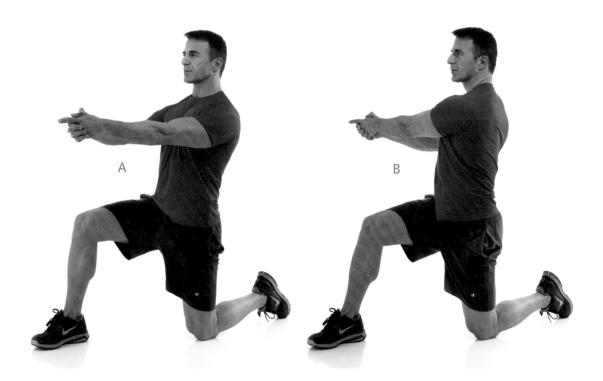

■ **C |** Switch the position of the legs, this time resting the right knee on the ground.

■ **D |** Now rotate arms and trunk to the left, again helping the movement by exhaling. Repeat for the same number of times.

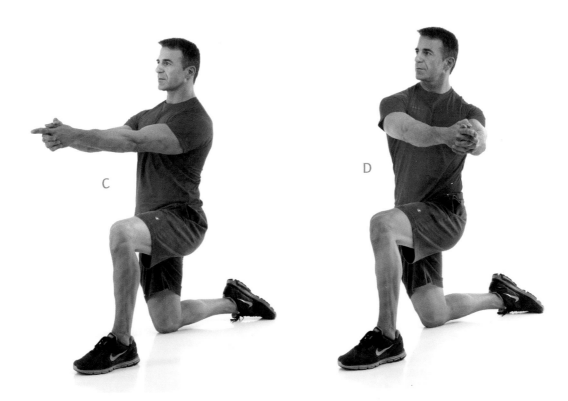

Discussion

I like exercises in the standing or half-kneeling position because the abdominal fascia is activated physiologically and functionally and you never lose touch with the world around you. The focus in the exercise isn't just the torso rotation that is controlled by the rectus abdominis, but it is also the destabilization induced by the upper body's rotation and by the acceleration imparted by its weight. These are comprehensive exercises. You may like them or you may not, but you should include them in any program.

KNEELING KILLER CRUNCH

Starting position

■ **A** | Adopt a kneeling position: the legs are flexed and the knees and feet are resting on the ground.
Extend the arms at chest height in front of your body and interlock the hands.

Execution

■ **B** | Exhaling, contract the rectus abdominis to stabilize the torso, and then rotate your arms and trunk fast to the right.

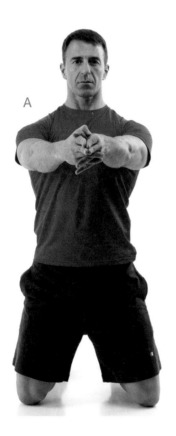

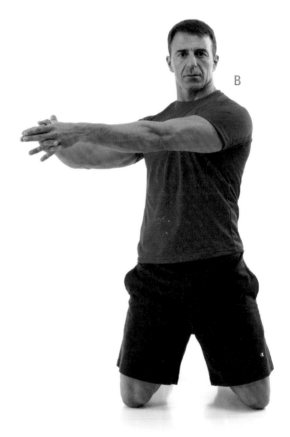

- **C** | Return to the center and perform 5-10 times.

- **D** | Repeat on the opposite side for the same number of repetitions.

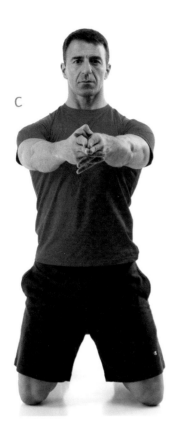

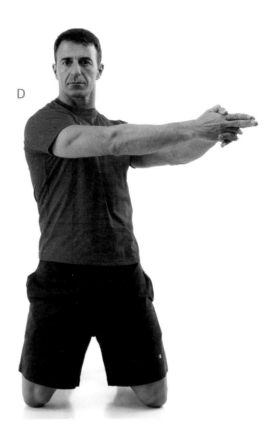

The kneeling position isolates the intervention of the muscles in the abdominal fascia and the hip to a greater degree. The action of the rectus abdominis is essential in this exercise to stabilize the trunk and protect the lumbar hinge. Equally important is the transversus and oblique muscles' activation, as they are dynamically involved in the exercise. As already underlined for the standing variation (standing killer crunch, p. 204), in this case the movement also ought to go beyond a simple twist, since this type of execution activates a nerve reflex, the myotatic reflex, which facilitates the action of the muscles involved. What you must do is rotate the trunk in one direction, return to the starting position, and repeat on the same side. Only when you have completed the number of required repetitions can you can move on to the opposite side.

10.6 UPPER-BODY EXERCISES

PUSH-UP

Starting position

- **A |** Adopt the plank position on your arms: Body in the prone position (belly down), straight as a plank.

Arms straight, resting on the hands at shoulders width.
Feet together, resting on the forefeet.

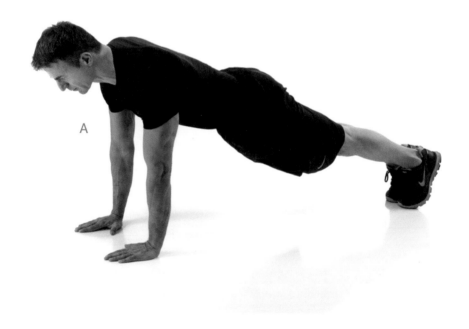

Execution

- **B** | Let your body fall slowly; the arms and elbows are close to the sides, the elbows turned backward.

Once on the ground, push the body upward, straightening the arms. Complete the required number of repetitions.

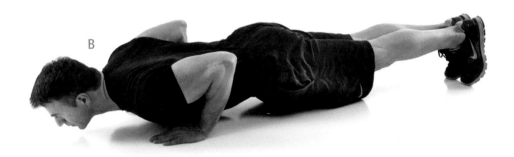

Discussion

Push-ups are a cult in the US. This exercise is often mistreated. In other words, it is badly executed, but it is exceptional for the upper part of the body. The key point is the position of the arms, which must be close to the torso both in the rising and descending phase. The most common mistakes in push-ups are:

- Calling them *flexions*; let me remind you that a flexion has no ground support.
- Executing them with arms wide; doing so causes greater stress on the upper back muscles, causing inflammation problems.
- Executing them partially, with an incomplete movement, which increases the kyphosis action of the pectoralis, the latissimus dorsi, and the anterior deltoid muscles.

With the push-up you will work more on the weak links of the kinematic chain involved—triceps and clavicular fascia of the pectoralis major—with no stress increase on joints and articular capsules and with no shortening of the pectoralis. Circle it in red.

SPIDER PUSH-UP

Starting position

- **A** | Lie in the prone position (belly down), with the hands just below the shoulders; arms and elbows are close to the sides.

Execution

- **B** | Push the body up by straightening the arms.

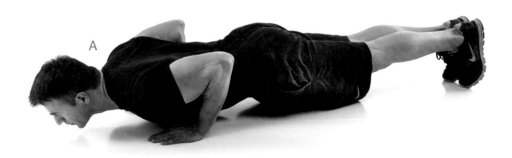

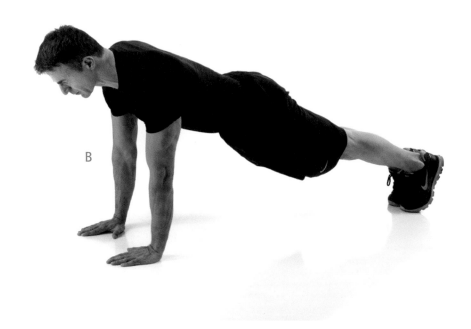

- **C |** As you descend, flex the left thigh laterally, bringing the knee close to the left arm.

- **D |** Rise again and repeat the push-up with the right thigh. Complete the required number of repetitions.

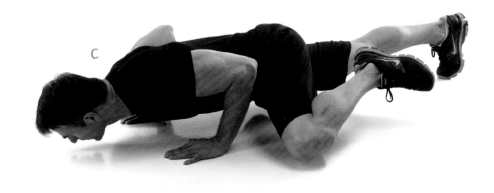

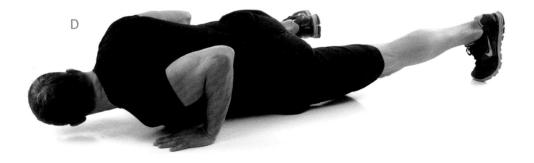

Discussion

We already saw how changing the position of the limbs modifies the effects of the exercise, because we engage other muscular systems which would be less stimulated otherwise. In the spider push-up, the change in the position of the lower body leads to a greater involvement of the core. This happens both in the stabilizing action and in the dynamic action, since the thigh's lateral flexion activates the oblique muscles, as flexors on one side and as stabilizers on the other. Equally, the destabilizing action increases the stimulus to the upper body alternately.

ALTERNATING LEGS PUSH-UP

Starting position

- A | Lie in the prone position (belly down), with the hands just below the shoulders; arms and elbows are close to the sides.

Execution

- B | Push the body up by straightening the arms.

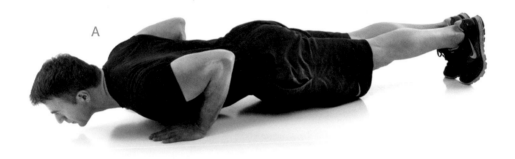

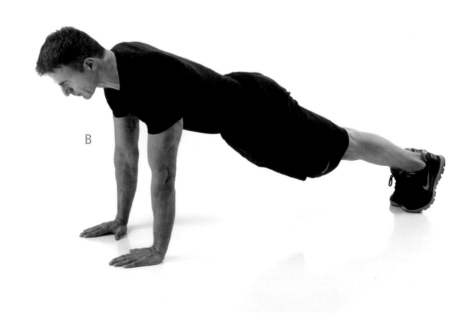

- **C |** As you descend, extend the left thigh up.
- **D |** Rise again and repeat the extension with the right thigh.

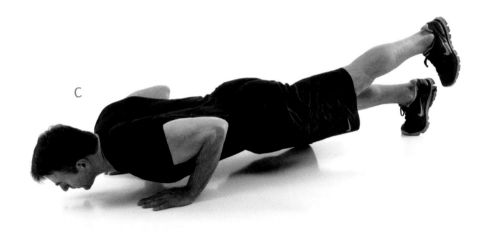

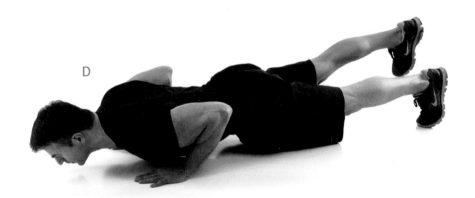

Discussion

The same that was said for the previous exercise is the same for this exercise. In this case there is a greater involvement of the core and the gluteus maximus.

CLOCK PUSH-UP

Starting position

- A | Lie in the prone position (belly down), with the hands just below the shoulders; arms and elbows are close to the sides.]

Execution

- B | Push the body up by straightening the arms.

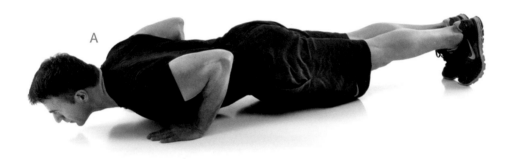

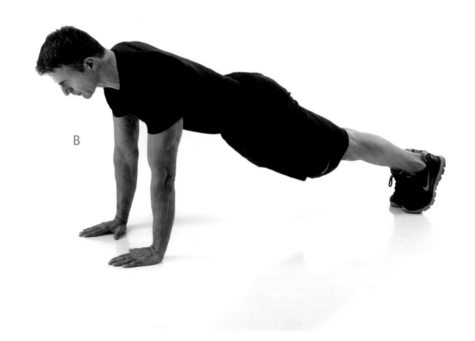

■ **C |** As you descend, abduct the left thigh, drawing it away from the other.

■ **D |** Rise up again and repeat the abduction with the right thigh.

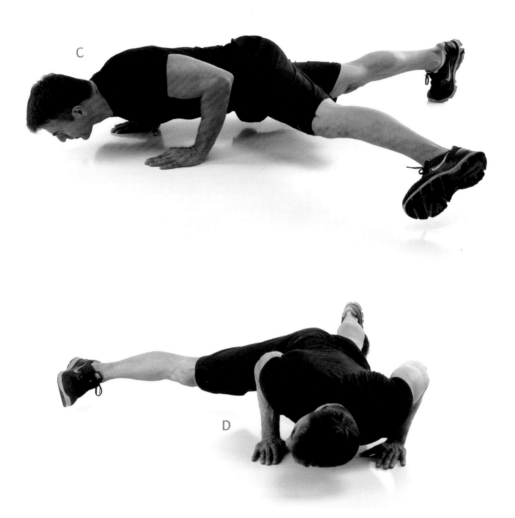

Discussion

This exercise is similar but not identical to the spider push-up (p. 222). In this exercise, the lateral flexion is carried out by the whole of the lower limb, a long lever, hence the lateral flexing action is decidedly more destabilizing. Essentially, the pectoralis, triceps, and oblique muscles are activated to a greater degree.

PLYOMETRIC PUSH-UP

Starting position

- **A |** Lie in the prone position (belly down), with the hands just below the shoulders; arms and elbows are close to the sides.

Execution

- **B |** Lower the body by bending the elbows, and then push the body upward explosively so that the hands and the upper body are suspended in the air for an instant, without touching the floor. Contact the ground again, stabilize the position, and re-start. Repeat for a maximum of 5 repetitions.

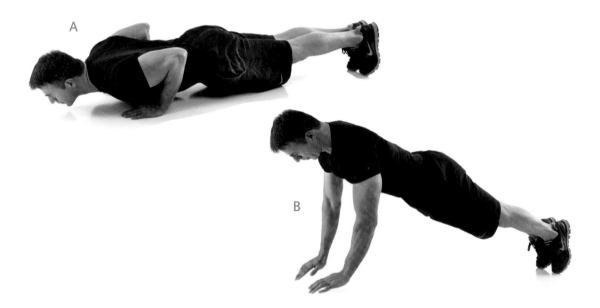

Discussion

Plyometric exercises have always been considered as the basis of athletic training for competitive sports. And also as one of the problems, if they are executed haphazardly or inserted in a training program at random. To begin with, they must not be approached recklessly by raising the torso too high or clapping the hands, for example, resulting in a hefty trauma to the wrist, elbow, and shoulder joints! Simply make a gentle initial effort as suggested in the exercise, just enough to raise up from the ground. Few exercises increase strength and power like plyometrics, but do them with caution.

BEAST PUSH-UP

Starting position

- **A |** Lie in the prone position (belly down), with the hands just below the shoulders; arms and elbows are close to the sides.

Execution

- **B |** Lower your body by bending the elbows, and then push your body forward and upward explosively, so as to throw yourself forward.

- **C |** Cushion the ground impact with the arms and return to the starting position. Prepare for the next explosive movement and perform the required number of repetitions, initially no more than 5.

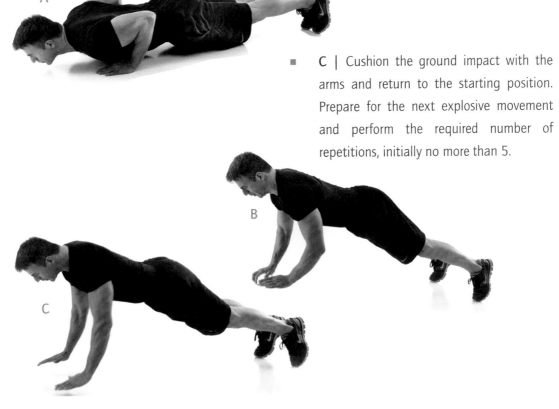

Discussion

This isn't an exercise for beginners, nor does it pretend to be. Very few people can perform the beast push-up. It is, of course, part of the training for wrestling and combat arts. This is a plyometric exercise to the nth power, so what was said for the previous exercise in terms of pros and cons is the same for this exercise.

LACERTA PUSH-UP

Starting position

- **A |** Lie prone on the ground (belly down). Raise your torso; the arms are straight, shoulders perpendicular to the hands, and legs lying on the ground.

Execution

- **B |** Start dragging your body along using only the arms.

- **C |** Bring first one arm then the other forward. Complete the distance required.

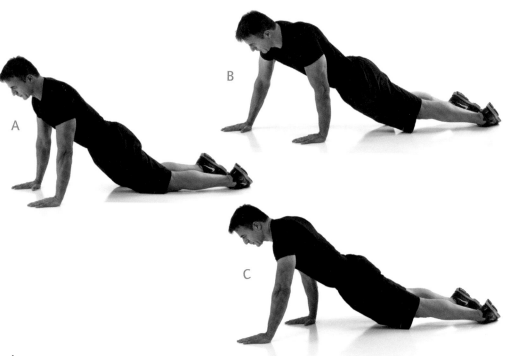

Discussion

One of the criticisms to free body-weight exercises is that there are no exercises which train the latissimus dorsi, unless you use a bar for pull-ups (something which isn't exactly for everyone, since it means lifting your body weight). Wrong! There are two exercises which train the latissimus dorsi and do it very well: the lacerta push-up and the floor pull (p. 242). Regarding the lacerta push-up, every time the trunk is suspended, both pectoralis and latissimus dorsi contribute synergistically to its stability. In summary: The pectoralis, latissimus dorsi, triceps, and deltoid muscles are fully stimulated by this innovative exercise, and you will soon notice it.

LEOPARD PUSH-UP

Starting position

- A | Lie in the prone position (belly down), with the hands just below the shoulders; arms and elbows are close to the sides.

Execution

- B | Push your body upward.

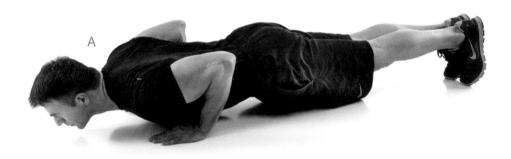

A

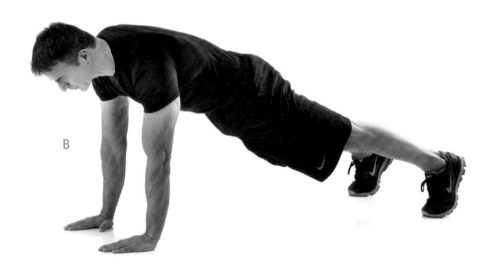

B

■ **C |** Move both right arm and left leg forward at the same time.

■ **D |** Lower your body down, keeping the arms close to the body as much as possible.

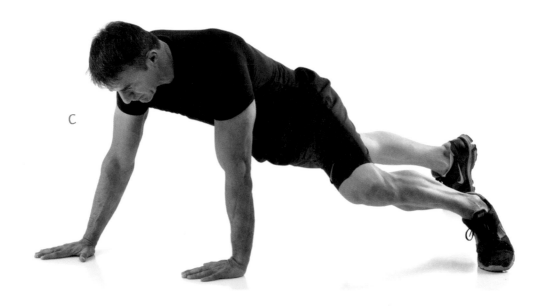

C

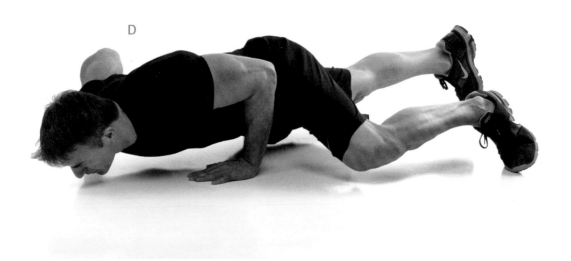

D

■ **E** | Now move the left arm and right leg forward at the same time.

■ **F** | Lower your body to the ground, still keeping the hands close to the body. Proceed this way, alternating legs and arms, for the required number of repetitions.

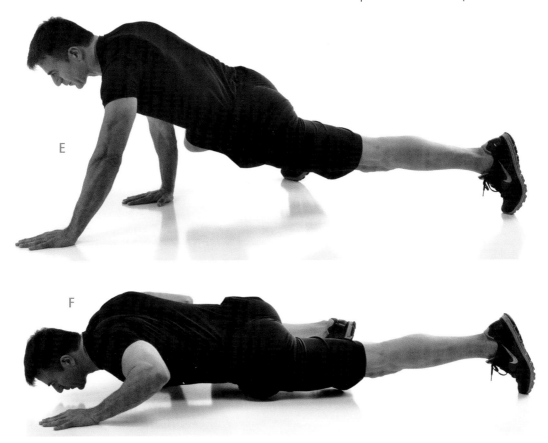

Discussion

This is a very comprehensive exercise for the whole body, not just the pectoralis muscle. The pectoralis muscle originates from a series of fixed digitations at the sternum, rib, and clavicle level; the distal insertion lies instead in the bicipital groove of the humerus, which is mobile. It is clear that the engagement of the various bands of the pectoralis muscle will depend on the position the humerus will take during the extension exercises. This is the reason why we train on inclined, level, and inverted benches in gyms. In the leopard push-up the position of the humerus varies from repetition to repetition; thus the whole pectoralis is involved in all its components. I would not underestimate the engagement of the latissimus dorsi, trapezius, triceps, and deltoid muscles.

ASYMMETRIC PUSH-UP

Starting position

- **A** | Lie in the prone position (belly down), with the hands just below the shoulders; arms and elbows are close to the sides.

Execution

- **B** | Raise up from the ground into the plank position.

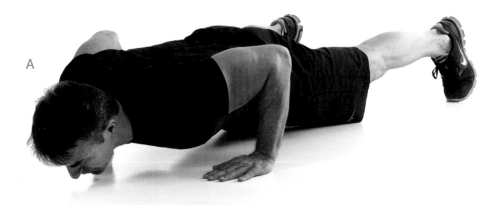

A

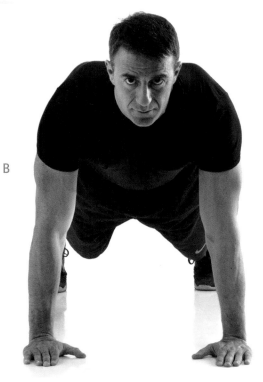

B

- **C |** Now bend your arms in a controlled fashion and descend, bringing the body toward the left arm. When you bring the weight toward an arm, there should be a sort of window between the opposite arm, the forearm, and the ground.

- **D |** Raise up again and repeat the exercise, bringing the weight toward the right arm.

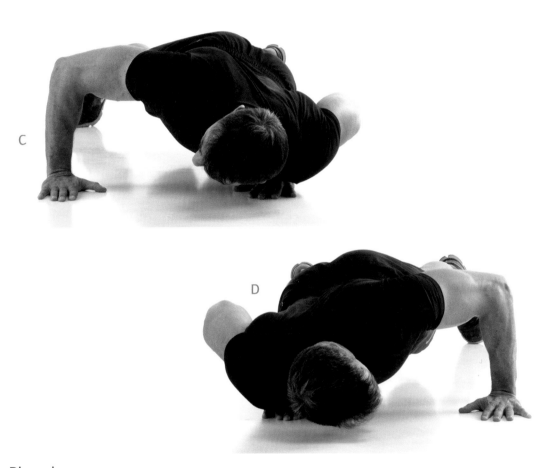

Discussion

If you vary the load from one side to the other, you stimulate to a greater degree the contractile activity in the pectoralis muscle of the arm toward which you are shifting the body and the stretching activity in that of the arm you are moving away from. This isn't an exercise for everyone, as the stress along the upper-back muscles isn't light. It is suitable for all contact sports such as combat arts, MMA, wrestling, rugby, and American football.

DYNAMIC SIDE PUSH-UP

Starting position

- A | Lie in the prone position (belly down), with the hands just below the shoulders; arms and elbows are close to the sides.

Execution

- B | Lift off the ground as if your body were one single plank.

- C | Shift to the right, crossing the left arm behind the right arm .

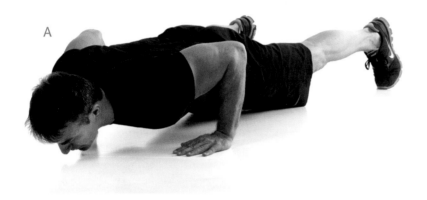

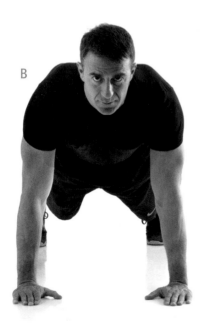

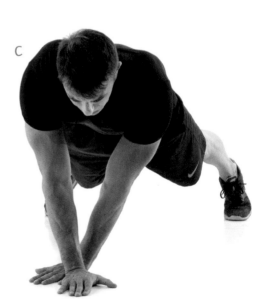

■ **D |** Shift the right arm to the right and execute a push-up.

■ **E |** Return to the starting position by crossing the right arm behind the left one and then shifting the left arm.

■ **F |** Shift to the left, crossing the right arm behind the left arm. Shift the left arm to the left and execute another push-up.

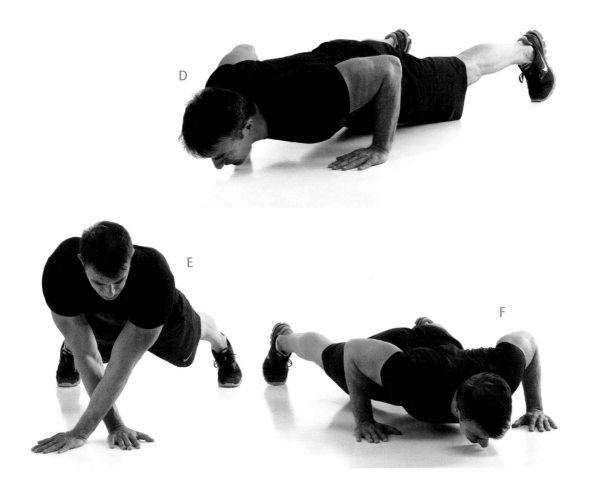

Discussion

This exercise is interesting. To a normal push-up, a chest-shoulders-torso stimulation, we add a crossover movement by changing direction. This implies an even greater activation of the pectoralis and also of the latissimus dorsi, which contributes to trunk stabilization. Add to this the engagement of the serratus muscle and the whole core, as well as the triceps and deltoid muscles.

DIAMOND PUSH-UP

Starting position

- **A** | Lie in the prone position (belly down), with the hands just below the shoulders; arms and elbows are close to the sides.
  Bring the hands close together, until thumb and index fingers of either are almost touching each other. The space between the hands looks like the shape of a diamond (hence the name of the exercise).
  Raise into plank position.

Execution

- **B** | Bend the arms, keeping the elbows close to the torso, and lower your body down. Don't stiffen your scapulae but, as you descend, let them follow the movement as they adduct.

- **C** | Rise up again by straightening the arms.

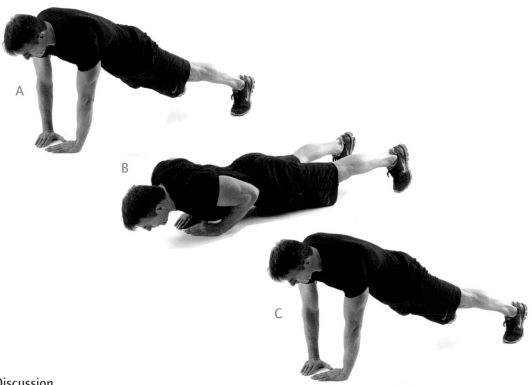

Discussion

This isn't an exercise for everyone. It requires mobility, especially in the wrist joint. But it is extremely effective. The stress is applied mainly to the triceps, pectoralis, trapezius, and rhomboid muscles.

BRAVE PUSH-UP PLYO CIRCUIT

Starting position

- **A |** Lie in the prone position (belly down), with the hands just below the shoulders; arms and elbows are close to the sides. Raise by straightening the arms.

Execution

- **B |** Bend the arms and lower your body again.

- **C |** Now begin this sequence: Extend the arms explosively; clap your hands during the brief aerial phase.

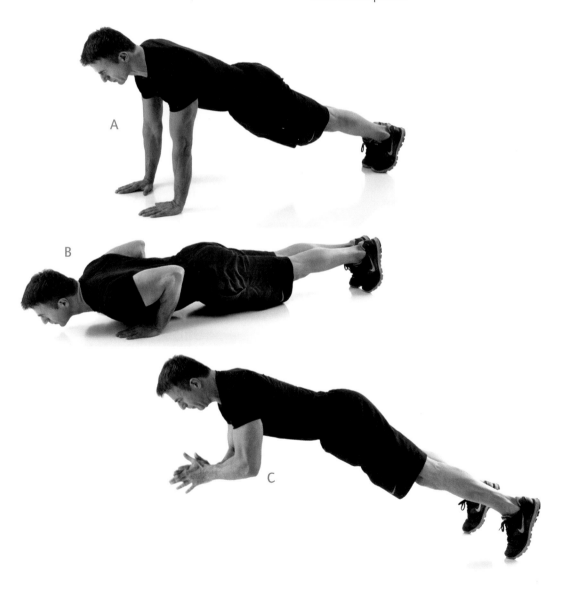

- **D |** Support yourself again; descend rapidly.

- **E |** Extend the arms explosively; strike the pectorals with both hands during the aerial phase.

- **F |** Support yourself again; descend rapidly.

- **G |** Extend the arms explosively; strike your

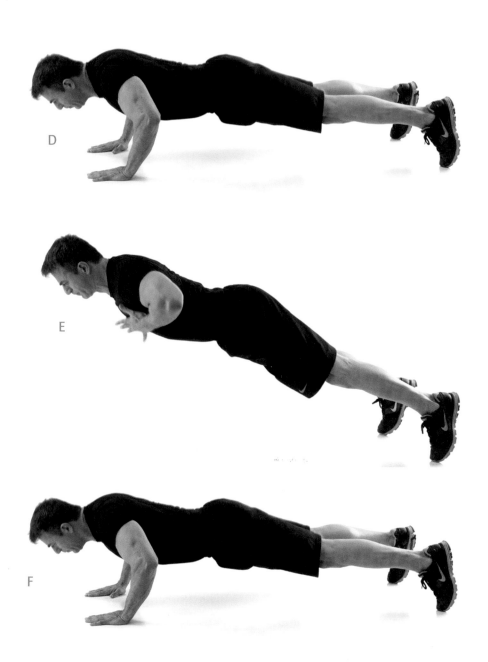

abdomen with both hands during the aerial phase.

■ **H |** Support yourself again; descend rapidly.

I | Extend the arms explosively; clap your hands behind your back by the lumbar area during the aerial phase. Support yourself again one last time.

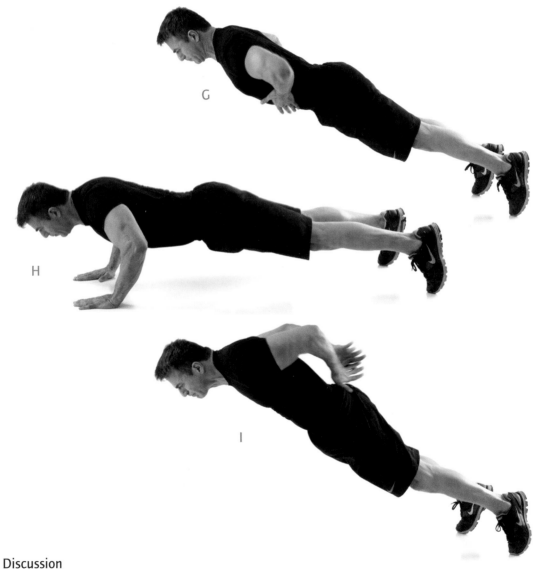

Discussion

There isn't much to discuss. This is a very tough plyometric circuit, for a few people only, but not that few. If you don't try...

FLOOR PULL

Starting position

■ **A** | Lie prone on the ground (belly down); support your body on the forearms, with the upper part of the torso raised.

Execution

■ **B** | Extend the arms forward, forming fists with your hands. Set the forearms on the ground and press the fists on the floor.

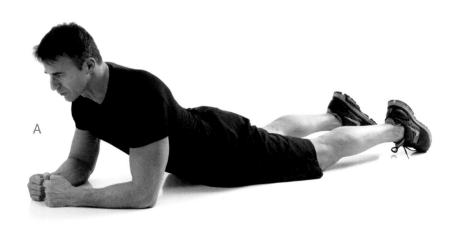

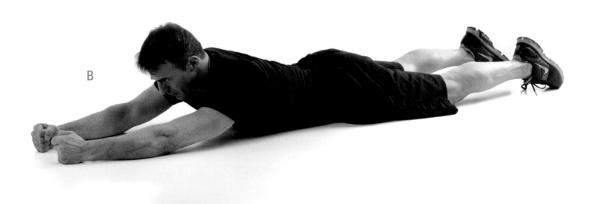

■ **C |** Using the wrists, pull the body forward. ■ **D |** Bring forearms and fists forward again, pulling yourself forward. Complete the repetitions or the distance required.

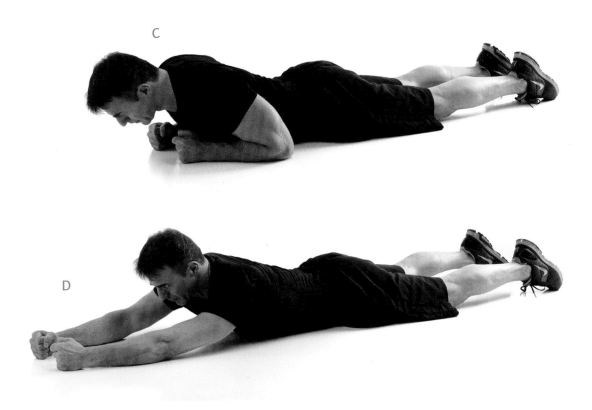

Discussion

One of the criticisms against body-weight exercises is that there aren't any exercises to train the latissimus dorsi, apart from bar pull-ups and their variations. This isn't true. There are at least two functional exercises: the lacerta push-up (p. 230) and the floor pull. This wonderful exercise, which I saw practiced by the great Martin Rooney, imitates a traction movement on the frontal plane (like the lat machine) and majorly activates the latissimus dorsi, pectoralis, trapezius, biceps muscles, and the long end of the triceps. My advice is to not extend the arms forward too much when starting—everyone will be able to perform it this way—but rather lengthen the lever gradually. More gains for the latissimus dorsi!

LARGE FLOOR PULL

Starting position

- **A |** Lie prone on the ground (belly down); support your body on the forearms, with the upper part of the torso raised.
  Close your hands into a fist.

Execution

- **B |** Extend the arms forward, keeping them about 20 in. away from one another. Set your forearms on the ground and press into the floor with the fists.

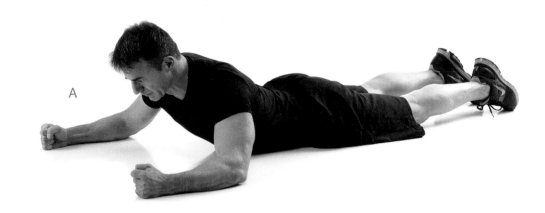

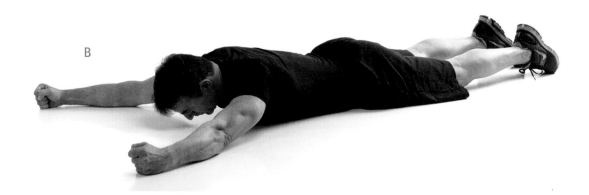

- **C |** Using the fists, pull your body forward.
- **D |** Bring forearms and fists forward again, and pulling yourself forward. Complete the repetitions or the distance required.

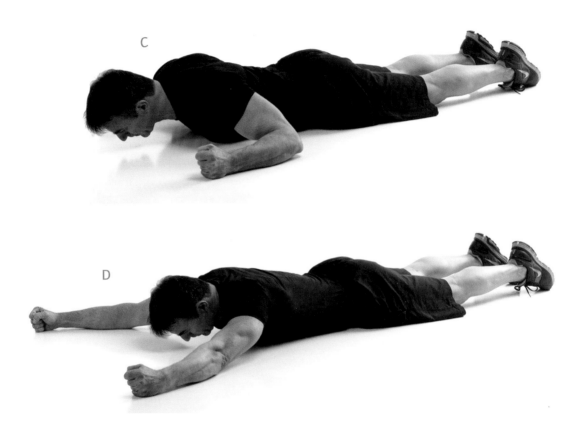

Discussion

This exercise is similar to the previous one. The arm adduction movement to the trunk is narrower than in the floor pull, but the lever is less advantageous. It will tend to activate the upper bands of the latissimus dorsi. There is, however, a different work angle. Remember that the latissimus dorsi is the human body's muscle with the largest surface, and, in order to train it comprehensively, we must combine exercises on the frontal plane to others on the sagittal plane. On both these planes, and those intermediate between them, we must work on several angles.

ALTERNATE FLOOR PULL

Starting position

- **A |** Lie down on the ground in the prone position (belly down); support your body on the forearms, with the upper part of the torso raised.
  Close your hands into a fist.

Execution

- **B |** Extend the right arm forward and set the forearm on the ground.

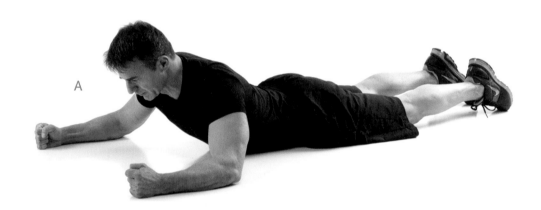

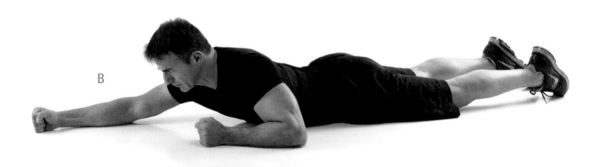

■ **C |** Using your right fist, pull the body forward and at the same time bring the left forearm forward.

■ **D |** Exerting pressure on the left fist, pull the body forward and bring forward the right forearm again. Repeat this sequence for the repetitions or distance required.

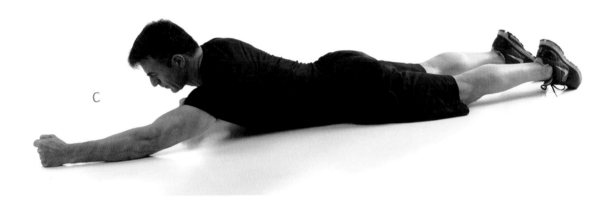

C

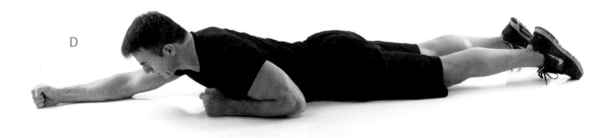

D

Discussion

Alternate work has a greater training effect on the latissimus dorsi, because the body's traction is borne entirely by one limb only.

FLOOR PRESS

Starting position

- **A** | Lie prone on the ground (belly down). Rest on the forearms, keeping them close to the trunk, and raise the upper part of the torso.

Execution

- **B** | Exert pressure on the ground with hands and forearms and, overcoming the resistance caused by your own weight, push the body backward, extending the arms gradually.

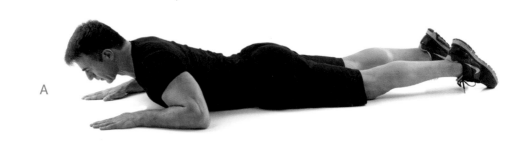

A

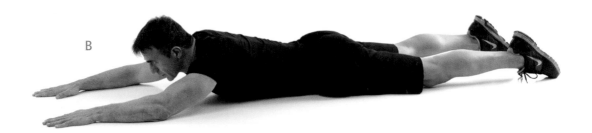

B

■ **C** | Bring the forearms and hands toward the chest again.

■ **D** | Push the body backward again. Complete the repetitions or the distance required.

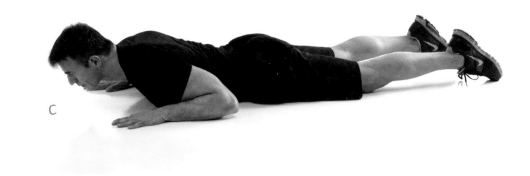

C

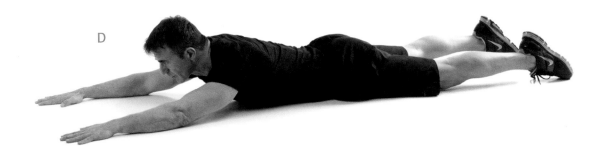

D

Discussion

The movement is the opposite to the floor pull (p. 242), and it is harder, because we are stronger in traction rather than extension movements by atavistic heredity. The exercise activates the antagonists of the muscles stimulated in the previous exercise, chiefly the deltoid and the triceps.

ALTERNATE FLOOR PRESS

Starting position

- **A |** Lie prone on the ground (belly down); support your body on the forearms, keeping them close to the trunk.

Execution

- **B |** Exert pressure on the ground with the left hand and forearm and push the body backward by extending them gradually.

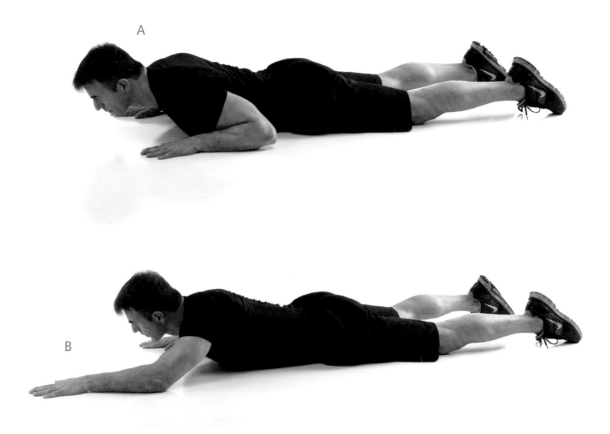

Discussion

This is tougher than the previous exercise, since only one arm at a time can overcome body-weight resistance. What was previously said therefore holds true...and doubly so!

■ **C |** Now apply the same force with right forearm, extending it and pushing the body backward again.

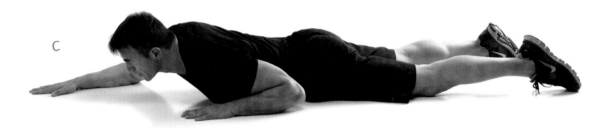

C

WALL PUSH-UP

Starting position	Execution

Starting position

■ Position close to a wall, the arms straight, the body raised, the feet resting on the wall behind you and exerting pressure.

Execution

■ Holding the starting position, bend the arms and descend with the torso and legs. Move your feet as if you were walking down the wall toward the ground.

■ Raise arms, torso, and legs together, moving the feet again upward with two small steps.

■ Complete the number of repetitions required.

Discussion

I have seen master Alberto Gallazzi perform this fantastic but tough exercise. The wall support is the key to the execution of the wall push-up and its effects. You will feel the core, the upper body, and the torso work like never before.

PART III – OBJECTIVES, METHODS, AND TRAINING PROGRAMS

CHAPTER

11

STRENGTH

11.1 THE FUNCTIONAL CHOICE

Your body as the best-fitting outfit; a new feeling of efficiency; and technical gestures once unthinkable now become easily-mastered exercises. If you have fully understood the concept of functional training, then maybe you are already feeling all this and experiencing it firsthand. You are only taking your first steps, yet you feel that something is changing, and more will change. I am now forced to dampen your enthusiasm, however, and remind you that functional training is a choice but not an excuse to throw away all you previously practiced in gyms. Actually, its first application is a return to basic exercises, suitably improved and adapted.

Action + Function = Functional training

We must not forget the importance of basic gym exercises such as squats, lunges, pulls, and presses. In this respect, and according to the definition I gave, the performance of weightlifting athletes in clean and jerk and snatch exercises is extremely functional. We have, in fact, an extremely powerful action of the hip extensor chain: a motor action first, then a stabilizing action by the abdominal fascia, and finally, these forces are conducted to the upper body. What do a boxer, a baseball player, a tennis player, and a golfer have in common? Apparently nothing, but if you observe the movement biomechanics, you will find the same concepts previously expressed: wind-up and activation of the hip extensor chain; motor and stabilizing action of the abdominal fascia; and transduction of these forces to the upper body. Have I made myself clear?

The following programs presented in chapters 11 through 13 include bonus exercises which use the following weights: kettlebells, medicine balls, and sandbags. As you progress in strength, you can transition from bodyweight to adding more weight by using the different equipment. For more details on performing the exercises, see the other volumes in The Ultimate Functional Training Series: *Training With Kettlebells, Training With Medicine Balls,* and *Training With Sandbags.*

11.2 STRENGTH TRAINING

We can define strength as the ability to defeat a resistance or to oppose it with a muscular effort (Zatziorskj).

Strength is a conditional ability, which depends about 80% on nerve factors. These factors imply:

- Maximum capacity for recruitment of type II white fibers (IIx especially).
- Maximum development of the central nervous system which, we may remember, takes place approximately by the age of 14.
- The ability to deactivate Renshaw's cells, the cells that act as breakers of the motor message.

The remaining 20% consists of organic and metabolic factors.

- The percentage of type IIa and type IIx white fibers.
- The density, hence the quantity, of white fibers within the transverse section area of the muscle.
- Increase in the diameter of white fibers.
- Improvements in recruitment (see chapter 5).

11.3 STRENGTH-TRAINING PROGRAMS

There are specific programs for strength training. The limit of the programs that follow is that they lack maximal tests and the work on the load percentages for those who pursue such objectives. I have therefore based mine on load progression and on increasing volume and workload by progressively higher-weight percentages within a "wave" program. The positive fact is that they work for everyone.

PROGRAM 1	
WORKOUT A	**WORKOUT B**
Run 10 min	Run 10 min
Squat 3 x 10.8.6 One-leg kettlebell deadlift 3 x 10 + 10	At-the-shoulder lunge with sandbag 3 x 10 + 10 Overhead squat with kettlebell 3 x 10 + 10
Deadlift 3 x 10.8.6 Pull-up 3 x max	Rower with two sandbags 3 x 10 Clean and press with two kettlebells 3 x 15
Horizontal bench press 3 x 10.8.6 Sandbag clean and press 3 x 15	Front shoulder press with barbell 3 x 10 Snatch with kettlebell 3 x 10
Run 10 min	Run 10 min

Training code
Total-body on major areas
Frequency: 2-3 times per week
Duration: 8-9 weeks
Note to workout A: Rotate the pairs of exercises every week so as to distribute the energies equally on all major areas.
Workout A progression: Every two weeks add a set of 6 to the first exercise in each group with a pyramidal method, up to a maximum of 5
Workout B progression: Every two weeks add 1 set to the first exercise in each listed pair.

PROGRAM 2	
WORKOUT A	**WORKOUT B**
Run 10 min	Run 10 min
Deadlift 4 x 8.6.6.4 Front squat 3 x 10.8.10	One-leg deadlift 3 x 10 One-leg squat 3 x 10
Horizontal bench press 4 x 8.6.6.4 Pull and press with sandbag 3 x 10	Clean and press with sandbag 3 x 20 Sandbag floor pull 3 x 20
Pull-up 4 x max Push press with two kettlebells 3 x 10	Push press with barbell 3 x 10 Tight grip bench 3 x 10
Run 10 min	Run 10 min

Training code
Total-body on major areas
Duration: 8 weeks
Frequency: 3 workouts per week
Notes to sheet A: Rotate the exercise pairs.

PROGRAM 3	
WORKOUT A	**WORKOUT B**
Run 10 min	Run 10 min
Horizontal bench press 5 x 5; recovery 4 min Low pulley 3 x 10; recovery 2 min	Dumbbell press on fitness ball 3 x 10; recovery 1 min 30 sec Clean and press with kettlebell 3 x 10
Squat 5 x 5 Leg curl on fitness ball 3 x 10	Pull-up 3 x max One-leg deadlift with two kettlebells 3 x 10, each side
Deadlift 5 x 5 Lat machine anterior 3 x 10	Barbell curl 3 x 10 Parallel dips 3 x max
Run 10 min	Run 10 min

Training code
Total-body
Duration: 8 weeks
Frequency: 3 times per week

PROGRAM 4	
WORKOUT A	**WORKOUT B**
Run 10 min	Run 10 min
Squat 3 x 7-9; 3 x 4-6; 3 x 11; recovery 4 min Swing with kettlebell 3 x 20 Military press 3 x 7-9 Clean with kettlebell 3 x 20 Narrow-grip bench press 3 x 7-9	Deadlift 3 x 7-9; 3 x 4-6; 3 x 11 Floor pull 3 x 20 One-leg deadlift 3 x 7-9 Walking lunge with rotation 3 x 10, each side Barbell curl 3 x 7-9
Run 10 min	Run 10 min

WORKOUT C
Run 10 min
Horizontal bench press 3 x 7-9; 3 x 5-7; 3 x 11 Floor press 3 x 20 Clean and press with kettlebell 3 x 7-9 Med ball side lunge with rotation 3 x 10, each side Snatch with kettlebell 3 x 20, each side
Run 10 min

PROGRAM 5	
WORKOUT A	**WORKOUT B**
Run 10 min	Run 10 min
Power swing with kettlebell 3 x 10 sec Squat 3 x 6; 3 x 3; 3 x 11 Pull-up 3 x max Push press with kettlebell 4 x 5-7 Barbell curl 3 x 10	Kneeling jump 3 x 5 Deadlift 3 x 6; 3 x 3; 3 x 9 Clean and press with kettlebell 3 x 5-7 One-leg deadlift 3 x 5-7 Crossover push-up 3 x 10
Run 10 min	Run 10 min

WORKOUT C
Run 10 min
Plyo push-up 3 x 5 Horizontal bench press 3 x 5; 3 x 3; 3 x 9 Low pulley 3 x 10 Leopard plank 3 x 20 Parallel dips 3 x max
Run 10 min

CHAPTER

12

HYPERTROPHY

12.1   HYPERTROPHY TRAINING

One whole book on this subject wouldn't be enough. There are one thousand and one studies on hypertrophy, but also no certainties as to the mechanism and the cause/effect of the hypertrophic stimulus. Just think about muscular fibers: They can be white, red, intermediate, totipotent, or satellite; each of these responds to one or more different stimuli. Not to mention the other components of the skeletal muscle: the sarcoplasmic, connective or lipid components, or that huge mystery that the brain still is today, with the cerebellum and nervous system, from which everything departs and where everything ends up. This gray area explains the profusion of techniques and methods, ranging from the scientific to the picturesque or the fanciful. Do we have to make do with what is available? Shall we continue with the approximations and anecdotal fantasies of odd guys in gyms? No, we shan't. We must understand our body, a perfect machine to which no computer, even the most advanced, can be remotely compared. Our body has always adapted according to the function for which it was created and has evolved in the course of millennia.

Let's see the priorities then:

1. Training the function of an articular system or a kinematic chain. Do you remember? The purpose, the reason for which that system or chain was built and created and has evolved to the present day.

2. Training the planes involved in the gestures and actions which relate to these systems and kinematic chains. What is the sense of training thighs and glutes with exercises on the frontal plane only (squats and deadlifts) if the hip extensor chain and the coxofemoral joint both share movement ranges on the sagittal and intermediate planes too?

3. Multijoint exercises: There are no monoarticular gestures in daily life.

4. Management and alternation of the loads (i.e., periodization) and the stress induced by them.

This is where I want to start from. I want to integrate an ordinary gym exercise program and its progression with exercises and modifications typical of functional training.

]

12.2   COSMETIC AND FUNCTIONAL HYPERTROPHY

As I mention in my book *Kettlebell* (Elika Publishers), a dispute is raging in the gym world, a feud which has developed as physical culture has shifted gradually from a performance sport—working on strength and its adaptations—to a sport with purely aesthetic features. The dispute is between cosmetic and functional hypertrophy. Cosmetic hypertrophy, as defined by American athletic coaches, is an increase in muscle mass for its own sake, with the objective of climbing on-stage or exhibiting a well-defined, muscular physique, with no performance purposes. Functional hypertrophy instead is an increase in muscle mass for performance purposes, meaning that it is combined with features such as strength, agility, power, and speed. Where does the main difference between these two cultural extremes lie? In workouts and their adaptations. In workouts we must combine classic basic exercises with functional exercises in order to stimulate different kinematic chains and different motor qualities and skills. As for adaptations, they are connected with functional hypertrophy and involve the central nervous system to a greater degree.

12.3 FUNCTIONAL HYPERTROPHY-TRAINING PROGRAMS

PROGRAM 1	
WORKOUT A	**WORKOUT B**
Run 8 min	Run 8 min
*Horizontal bench press 3 x 10; recovery 2 min Push-up 3 x max; recovery 1 min 30 sec	*Horizontal bench dumbbell press 3 x 10 Leopard push-up 3 x 10
*Front lat machine (without knee pad) 3 x 10 Floor pull 3 x 10	*Rower with sandbag 3 x 10-15 Lacerta push-up 3 x 10
Barbell push press 3 x 10-12	*Squat jump 3 x 5 Walking lunge & rotation 3 x 5 each side
*Front squat 3 x 10 Walking lunge 3 x 10, each side	Frontal stabilizers on forearms 3 x 10 sec Reverse crunch with sandbag 3 x 10
Straight-arm front stabilizers 3 x 10 sec Oblique crunches 3 x 10, each side	Run 8 min
Run 8 min	

Training code
Total-body
Duration: 6-8 weeks
Progression: every week add 1 set to the exercises marked by *

PROGRAM 2	
WORKOUT A	**WORKOUT B**
Run 8 min	Run 8 min
Horizontal bench press 3 x 10.8.6; recovery 2 min Leopard push-up 3x10, each side; recovery 1 min 30 sec	*Push-up on kettlebells 3 x max Barbell push on fitness ball 3 x 10
Lat machine middle grip (without knee pad) 3 x 10.8.6 Rower with two sandbags 3 x 10, each side	*Sandbag floor pull 3 x 10 Rower with two kettlebells 3 x 10
	Sandbag clean and press 3 x 10
*Clean and press with two kettlebells 3 x 10 Diagonal press with med ball 3 x 10, each side	*Squat and press with kettlebell 3 x 10 One-leg kettlebell deadlift 3 x 10, each side
*Front squat with barbell 3 x 10 Walking lunge with rotation 3 x 10, each side	Side plank with rotation 5 x 10, each side
Run 8 min	Run 8 min

Training code
Total-body
Duration: 6-8 weeks
Progression: every 2 weeks add 1 set to the exercises marked by * (add 1 set of 6 reps to the exercises with pyramidal method)

PROGRAM 3	
WORKOUT A	**WORKOUT B**
Run 8 min	Pull-up 3 x max
*Front squat 3 x 5 At-the-shoulder lunge with sandbag 3 x 10, each side Power swing 3 x 10	*Reverse row: horizontal tractions from the multipower bar 3 x max Lacerta push-up 3 x 20
Plyo push-up 3 x 5-7 *Horizontal bench press 3 x 5 Push-up 3 x 10	*Double jerk with two kettlebells 3 x 5-7 Diagonal press with med ball 3 x 10, each side Bent press 3 x 7, each side
Barbell curls from the preacher position (kneeling on a mat, the pelvis off the heels) 3 x 7-9	Parallel dips 3 x max
Sandbag reverse crunch 3 x 10 Side plank 3 x 10 sec, each side	Leopard plank 3 x 30 sec Reverse rope crunch 3 x 10
Run 8 min	Run 8 min

Training code
Split routine
Duration: 6-8 weeks
Progression: every 2 weeks add 1 set to the exercises marked by *

PROGRAM 4	
WORKOUT A	**WORKOUT B**
Rope skipping 5 min	Run 10 min
Walking lunge with barbell 3 x 5, each side	Bent press with kettlebell 3 x 7, each side
Front squat and press 3 x 7-9	Pull-up 3 x max
Burpee 3 x 20	Sandbag floor pull 3 x 10
Dumbbell push 3 x 5	Clean and jerk with two kettlebells 3 x 7
Leopard push-up 3 x 20	Push press with kettlebell 3 x 15
Narrow-grip bench press 3 x 5	Barbell curl 3 x 5-7
Reverse rope crunch 3 x 20	Leopard plank 3 x 30 sec
Side plank with rotation 3 x 10, each side	Side plank with twist 3 x 10, each side
Rope skipping 5 min	Run 10 min

Training code

Split routine

Duration: 6-8 weeks

Progression: every week add 1 set to the first exercise for each muscle group, up to a maximum of 5 sets

SLIMMING

13.1 SLIMMING TRAINING

Those who follow me know that slimming is a metabolic condition with several "parents". There are many organic lipolytic paths, meaning there are different methods to start losing body fat. First of all let's clarify what we mean by slimming. We don't simply mean a decrease in weight. Scales are of little use in *slimming* (greatly overweight subjects excepted), because they don't measure the real decrease in body-fat percentage.

How to define slimming then? *Slimming* is a decrease in the lipid organic fractions, especially the subcutaneous and visceral ones. Let me start with a commonplace observation we should, however, keep in mind: There is no slimming without a suitable eating regimen, or at least it is extremely difficult. This point may appear obvious, but it happens to be the basic reason for a lack of results. Having said this, let me be clear that circuit work is suitable for other types of adaptations, too, from hypertrophy to strength. The neurogenic and muscular components involved are determined by the type of training stimulus.

13.2   LIPOLYTIC PATHS

Here is a brief review of the training stimuli to be "administered" (that term isn't chosen at random) to activate different lipolytic paths:

1.   Muscle tone training

Muscle tone is a very low-intensity electrical message that is always present in any active muscle, even at rest. This is typically a nerve adaptation, which can be reached by classic strength training. Strength training increases muscle tone over time; this generates an increase in the subject's basal metabolism and an increase in the oxidative work on body fats when at rest, too.

2.   Training for hypertrophy

Many people ask me what hypertrophy and slimming have in common. When completing an exercise to exhaustion, lactate production indicates a hormonal response by

- the growth hormone: proteolytic and lipolytic response;
- catecholamines: adrenaline and noradrenalin (lipolytic response); and
- thyroid hormones: lipolytic response.

But is this enough? There is actually more to this; for example, we know that by doing interval work up to the lactate threshold, we influence EPOC heavily. All this translates in a metabolic increase which lasts for several hours after training (depending on the intensity of the exercise, up to 12, 16, even 24 hours and more) with a 10-15% increase in body-fat burning at rest!

3.   Aerobic training

The oxidative paths in Krebs cycle are essential in providing the amount of oxygen necessary for lipolysis. Low-intensity aerobic work is indispensable for obese or greatly overweight subjects in the initial phase of training. It is important for beginners, too, though over time the intensity will have to increase progressively, reaching interval training and circuits. Regarding circuits, cardio-fit training, peripheral heart action, and circuit training methods are particularly beneficial.

Further progressions of these are:

- Blitz circuits, for their ability to put all organic systems under heavy stress in a very short time, reaching oxygen debt immediately.
- Timed circuits, for the efficient management of the gesture or gestures being performed.

13.3 CIRCUIT TRAINING

I have been talking about circuit training as the training for the future for at least a decade. You can stimulate highly differentiated systems and organic structures with one single method. Circuit training is essential for general physical preparation for any performance sports-specific training, for strength and hypertrophy training, and for creating a slimming strategy for everyone. The method variations make this a highly diverse type of training, never boring and with a level of intensity ranging from beginners to athletes. The best-known methods are circuit training, cardio-fit training, PHA training, Blitz circuits, timed circuits, and boot camp. Let's take a look at them.

13.3.1 Circuit training

Organized by the US Army around 1956, circuit training consists of a sequence of exercises, varying from 6 to 10 or more, to be repeated with little or no rest between each of them. The execution of one entire sequence of exercises is called a circuit. At the end of each circuit, you can choose between passive or active recovery before starting again.

The number of circuit runs varies from 2 to 10.

PROGRAM 1	PROGRAM 2
TOTAL-BODY PROGRAM FOR EVERYONE	FOR BEGINNER WOMEN
Run 10 min	Run 10 min
Push-up 1 x 10 Crunch 1 x 10 Clean with sandbag 1 x 10 Arms plank 1 x 10 min Walking lunge 1 x 10	Swing with kettlebell 1 x 20 Push-up 1 x 5-10 Walking lunge 1 x 5, 10, each side Arms plank 1 x 10 sec Squat and press with kettlebell 1 x 5/10
Reverse rope crunch 1 x 10 Recovery 2 min	Clean and press with sandbag 1 x 10 Walk 2 min
Repeat the sequence 5 times	Repeat the sequence 3-5 times
Run 10 min	Run 10 sec

PROGRAM 3	PROGRAM 4
FOR BEGINNER MEN	**FOR BEGINNER MEN**
Run 10 min	Run 10 min
Push-up 1 x 10 Rope crunch 1 x 10 Floor pull 1 x 10 Forearm plank 1 x 10 sec Front squat 1 x 10 Reverse rope crunch 1 x 10 Rower with sandbag 1 x 10 Leopard plank 1 x 10 sec Recovery 2 min Repeat the sequence 5 times Run 10 min	Leopard plank 1 x 10 Plyo push-up 1 x 5 Reverse rope crunch 1 x 10 Clean and press with kettlebell 1 x 10 Side plank with twist 1 x 10, each side Squat and press with kettlebell 1 x 10 Swing 1 x 20 Recovery 2 min Repeat the sequence 5 times Run 10 min

PROGRAM 5	PROGRAM 6
DYNAMIC EXERCISES FOR BEGINNER WOMEN	**DYNAMIC EXERCISES FOR BEGINNER MEN**
Run 10 min	Run 10 min
Jumping jack 1 x 10 Skip 1 x 10 sec Swing 1 x 10 Squat and press 1 x 10 Rope crunch 1 x 10 Push press with kettlebell 1 x 10 Sandbag reverse crunch 1 x 10 Clean and press with sandbag 1 x 10 Recovery 2 min Repeat the sequence 3-5 times Run 10 min	Skip 1 x 10 min Push-up 1 x 10 Jumping jack 1 x 10 Clean and press with sandbag 1 x 10 Burpee 1 x 10 Squat and press with kettlebell 1 x 10 Sandbag reverse crunch 1 x 10 Recovery 2 min Repeat the sequence 3-5 times Run 10 min

PROGRAM 7	PROGRAM 8
FOR INTERMEDIATE MEN	**FOR INTERMEDIATE WOMEN**
Swing 1 x 20	Run 10 min
Leopard push-up 1 x 20	Swing 1 x 20
Side plank with twist 1 x 10, each side	At-the-shoulder walking lunge with sandbag 1 x 10, each side
Burpee 1 x 20	Clean and press with kettlebell 1 x 10
Pull and press with sandbag 1 x 20	Swing 1 x 20
At-the-shoulder walking lunge with sandbag 1 x 10, each side	Burpee1 x 20
Side plank 1 x 10 sec, each side	Floor pull 1 x 20
Recovery 2 min	Reverse rope crunch 1 x 20
Repeat the sequence 5 times	Push press 1 x 10
Run 10 min	Recovery 2 min
	Repeat the sequence 3-5 times
	Run 10 min

PROGRAM 9	PROGRAM 10
FOR ADVANCED MEN	**FOR ADVANCED WOMEN**
Swing 7 min (alternate one-armed and two-armed)	Swing 7 min
Burpee 1 x 20	Burpee 1 x 20
Push-up with two kettlebells 1 x 20	Leopard plank 1 x 20
Med ball side lunge with rotation 1 x 10, each side	Push-up 1 x max
Leopard plank 1 x 20	At-the-shoulder lunge with rotation 1 x 10, each side
Pull-up 1 x 20	Side plank with rotation 1 x 5, each side
Squat and press with kettlebell 1 x 10-20	Clean and press with kettlebell 1 x 10-20
Rower with sandbag 1 x 20	Squat and press with kettlebell 1 x 10
Side plank with rotation 1 x 5, each side	Reverse rope crunch 1 x 20
Recovery 2 min	Rower with sandbag 1 x 20
Repeat the sequence 5 times	Recovery 2 min
Swing 7 min	Repeat the sequence 3-5 times
	Swing 7 min

13.3.2   Cardio-fit training

Cardio-fit training is a circuit training method that alternates aerobic phases—on cardio machines or with aerobic exercises (running, rope skipping, walking)—and anaerobic phases. Initially, the cardio phase is used as active recovery after an exercise phase. The circuit's level of difficulty is increased gradually, heightening the intensity of both the anaerobic and the aerobic phases. Cardio-fit training is a typical interval training method. This is its main strength.

In 1998 it was the subject of a study carried out by Neri, Paoli, and Velussi, who compared its slimming effects to those of the classic method of aerobic training. In the course of the study, they selected two groups of athletes, both composed of beginners. The first group trained on cardio machines only, while the second group performed cardio-fit training with triceps and abs exercises only. The plicometer test results were rather surprising: the degree of slimming in both groups was similar but on triceps and abs the cardio-fit group slimmed down twice as much! At a time when the diatribe on localized slimming was at its peak, the study had a lot of recognition and was the basis for a series of further studies which confirmed its results.

PROGRAM 1	PROGRAM 2
FOR BEGINNER WOMEN	FOR BEGINNER MEN
Cardio 10 min	Cardio 10 min
Squat 1 x 5 Lateral clean (quadrupedal) 1 x 10, each side Repeat 2 times without stopping	Push-up 1 x 10 Rope crunch 1 x 10 Repeat 2-3 times without stopping
Cardio 5 min	Cardio 5 min
Step-up 1 x 5, each side Backward clean (quadrupedal) 1 x 10, each side Repeat 2 times without stopping	Squat 1 x 5-7 Straight-arm stabilization 1 x 10 sec Repeat 2-3 times without stopping
Cardio 5 min	Cardio 5 min
Press with med ball 1 x 10 Straight-arm stabilization 1 x 10 sec Repeat 3 times without stopping	Press with sandbag 1 x 10 Rope diagonal crunch 1 x 5, each side Repeat 2-3 times without stopping
Cardio 5 min Rower with sandbag 1 x 10 Rope crunch 1 x 10 Repeat 3 times without stopping	Cardio 5 min Floor pull 1 x 10 Forearm stabilization 1 x 10 sec Repeat 2-3 times without stopping
Cardio 10 min	Cardio 10 min

PROGRAM 3	PROGRAM 4
FOR INTERMEDIATE WOMEN	**FOR INTERMEDIATE MEN**
Cardio 10 min	Cardio 10 min
Squat jump 1 x 5 Reverse rope crunch 1 x 10 Repeat 3 times without stopping	Med ball crossover push-up 1 x 6, each side Reverse rope crunch 1 x 10 Repeat 3 times without stopping
Cardio 5 min	Cardio 5 min
One-leg kettlebell deadlift 1 x 5, each side Box squat 1 x 5 Repeat 3 times without stopping	Clean and press with sandbag 1 x 10 Side plank with twist 1 x 10, each side Repeat 3 times without stopping
Cardio 5 min	Cardio 5 min
Floor pull 1 x 10 Side plank with twist 1 x 5, each side Repeat 3 times without stopping	Walking lunge 1 x 10, each side Side plank with rotation 1 x 5, each side Repeat 3 times without stopping
Cardio 5 min	Cardio 5 min
Med ball diagonal press 1 x 10, each side Reverse rope crunch 1 x 10 Repeat 3 times without stopping	Rower with two sandbags 1 x 10 Rope diagonal crunch 1 x 10, each side Repeat 3 times without stopping
Cardio 10 min	Cardio 10 min

PROGRAM 5	
FOR ADVANCED WOMEN	
Run 10 min	Cardio 5 min
Kettlebell overhead walking lunge 1 x 10, each side Lateral clean (quadrupedal) 1 x 10, each side Repeat 3 times without stopping	Clean and press with sandbag 1 x 10 Push-up 1 x 10 Repeat 3 times without stopping
Cardio 5 min	Cardio 5 min
Lu.Be.Lu.Be. 1 x 2 rounds, alternating Kettlebell swing 1 x 20 Repeat 3 times without stopping	Floor pull 1 x 15 Side plank with rotation 1 x 5, each side Repeat 3 times without stopping
	Cardio 10 min

PROGRAM 6	
FOR ADVANCED MEN	
Run 10 min	Cardio 5 min
Burpee 1 x 10 Leopard crunch 1 x 10, each side Repeat 4 times without stopping	Clean and press with two kettlebells 1 x 10 Squat and press with two kettlebells 1 x 10 Repeat 4 times without stopping
Cardio 5 min	Run 10 min
Sandbag floor pull 1 x 20 Plyo push-up 1 x 7 Repeat 4 times without stopping	

PROGRAM 7	PROGRAM 8
GENERAL PHYSICAL PREPARATION FOR WOMEN	**GENERAL PHYSICAL PREPARATION FOR MEN**
Run 10 min	Run 10 min
Swing 1 x 20 Squat and press with two kettlebells 1 x 10 Repeat 4 times without stopping	Leopard push-up 1 x 20 Sandbag floor pull 1 x 20 Repeat 4 times without stopping
Cardio 5 min	Cardio 3 min
Clean and press with sandbag 1 x 15 Rower with sandbag 1 x 15 Repeat 4 times without stopping	Med ball half-kneeling position with rotation 1 x 10, each side Side plank with rotation 1 x 10, each side Repeat 4 times without stopping
Cardio 5 min	Cardio 3 min
Push-up 1 x 10 Side plank with rotation 1 x 7, each side Repeat 4 times without stopping	Kettlebell squat and press 1 x 10 One-leg kettlebell deadlift 1 x 10, each side Repeat 4 times without stopping
Cardio 5 min	Cardio 3 min
Burpee 1 x 10 Rope V-crunch 1 x 10, each side Repeat 4 times without stopping	Rower with sandbag 1 x 20 Kettlebell renegade row 1 x 10, each side Repeat 4 times without stopping
Run 10 min	Run 10 min

13.3.3 Peripheral heart action (PHA) training

Created as a bodybuilding technique by Bob Gajda, PHA training has been subsequently applied to circuit training, as a method within the method. It can be applied to all the circuit training programs we have seen so far. It consists of an alternation of selected exercises, working on muscular areas distant from one another.

The distance between the areas stimulates the cardiorespiratory and cardiovascular systems strongly, increasing their activity. Their job is to provide oxygen and metabolites (which are then removed) to the muscles during the exercise. The lipolytic effect is decidedly greater.

Here are some examples of PHA training.

PROGRAM 1	PROGRAM 2
FOR BEGINNER WOMEN	FOR BEGINNER WOMEN
Cardio 10 min	Cardio 10 min
Squat 1 x 10 Med ball press 1 x 10 Repeat 3 times without stopping	Swing 1 x 20 Squat and press 1 x 10 Repeat 3 times without stopping
Cardio 5 min	Cardio 5 min
Walking lunge 1 x 5, each side Floor pull 1 x 10 Repeat 3 times without stopping	At-the-shoulder walking lunge with sandbag 1 x 10, each side Push-up 1 x 10 Repeat 3 times without stopping
Cardio 5 min	Cardio 5 min
Push-up with knee support 1 x 5 Rope V-crunch 1 x 5, each side Repeat 3 times without stopping	Kettlebell push press 1 x 10 One-leg kettlebell deadlift 1 x 10, each side Repeat 3 times without stopping
Cardio 5 min	Cardio 5 min
Kettlebell swing 1 x 10 Straight-arm plank 1 x 10 sec Repeat 3 times without stopping	Rower with sandbag 1 x 15 Reverse rope crunch 1 x 10 Repeat 3 times without stopping
Cardio 10 min	Cardio 10 min

PROGRAM 3	PROGRAM 4
FOR BEGINNER MEN	FOR BEGINNER MEN
Cardio 10 min	Cardio 10 min
Squat 1 x 10 Push-up 1 x 10 Repeat 3 times without stopping	At-the-shoulder sandbag squat 1 x 10, each side Med ball crossover push-up 1 x 7, each side Repeat 3 times without stopping
Cardio 5 min	Cardio 5 min
Floor pull 1 x 10 One-leg kettlebell deadlift 1 x 10, each side Repeat 3 times without stopping	Sandbag floor pull 1 x 20 At-the-shoulder sandbag lunge 1 x 10, each side Repeat 3 times without stopping
Cardio 5 min	Cardio 5 min
Med ball diagonal press 1 x 10, each side Plank 1 x 10 sec Repeat 3 times without stopping	Rower with two sandbags 1 x 20 Reverse rope crunch 1 x 15 Repeat 3 times without stopping
Cardio 5 min	Cardio 5 min
Burpee 1 x 5 Rope crunch 1 x 10 Repeat 3 times without stopping	One-leg kettlebell deadlift 1 x 10 Forearm plank 1 x 20 sec Repeat 3 times without stopping
Cardio 10 min	Cardio 10 min

PROGRAM 5	
FOR INTERMEDIATE WOMEN	
Run 10 min	Cardio 5 min
Burpee 1 x 10 Leopard plank 1 x 10, each side Repeat 3 times without stopping	Swing 1 x 30 Reverse rope crunch 1 x 20 Repeat 3 times without stopping
Cardio 5 min	Cardio 5 min
At-the-shoulder sandbag lunge 1 x 10, each side Push-up 1 x 10 Repeat 3 times without stopping	Sandbag floor pull 1 x 20 Med ball diagonal press 1 x 10, each side Repeat 3 times without stopping
	Cardio 10

PROGRAM 6
FOR INTERMEDIATE MEN

Run 10 men	Cardio 5 min
Swing 1 x 30 Double jerk 1 x 15 Repeat 3 times without stopping	Sandbag floor pull 1 x 20 Burpee 1 x 20 Repeat 3 times without stopping
Cardio 5 min	Cardio 5 min
Kettlebell squat and press 1 x 20 Med ball crossover push-up 1 x 10, each side Repeat 3 times without stopping	Side plank with twist 1 x 10, each side Kneeling jump 1 x 10 Repeat 3 times without stopping
	Run 10 min

PROGRAM 7	PROGRAM 8
FOR ADVANCED WOMEN	FOR ADVANCED MEN
Run 10 min	Run 10 min
Squat and press 1 x 10 Leopard plank 1 x 10, each side Repeat 3 times without stopping	Kettlebell squat and press 1 x 20 Leopard plank 1 x 20 Repeat 3 times without stopping
Run 5 min	Run 5 min
Lunge jump 1 x 7, each side Clean and press with sandbag 1 x 20 Repeat 3 times without stopping	Burpee 1 x 20 Leopard push-up 1 x 20 Repeat 3 times without stopping
Run 5 min	Run 5 min
Squat jump 1 x 5 Plyo push-up 1 x 5 Repeat 3 times without stopping	Kneeling jump 1 x 10 Side plank with rotation 1 x 10, each side Repeat 3 times without stopping
Run 5 min	Run 5 min
Med ball diagonal press 1 x 10, each side Reverse rope crunch 1 x 15 Repeat 3 times without stopping	Sandbag floor pull 1 x 20 Plyo push-up 1 x 10 Repeat 3 times without stopping
Run 10 min	Run 10 min

13.3.4   Blitz circuits

Widespread test evidence suggests we should bear in mind the following factors as the keys to reaching different objectives.

SLIMMING

1. Gradual work on EPOC is essential; increases in EPOC are related to the intensity of the exercise rather than its duration.
2. Increase in metabolic "horse power" through an increase in lean mass; the lean mass increase is chiefly promoted by lactacid work.
3. Muscle tone work; muscle tone increase (a much underestimated concept) is connected to alactacid training.
4. Lipolytic hormones activation (GH, testosterone, catecholamines, thyroid hormones) through lactacid–alactacid work.

TONING

1. Lean mass increase.
2. Muscle tone increase.
3. Anabolic hormones activation (GH, IGF-1, IGF-2, testosterone, FGF, insulin) through lactacid–alactacid work.
4. Training should concentrate exclusively on alactacid–lactacid workouts.

Starting from these premises I have developed blitz training circuits that are fast, intense, and effective. They last up to 30 min, and this is more than enough! Blitz circuit effectiveness is related to its intensity; basic exercise selection will be key, as well as the loads, which will point in the direction of the desired objective (slimming, toning, muscle tone, or hypertrophy).

PROGRAM 1	PROGRAM 2
SLIMMING	**SLIMMING FOR WOMEN**
Cardio 5 min: ideally walking, (stationary) steps, running, horizontal bike	Cardio 5 min: ideally walking, (stationary) steps, running, horizontal bike
Dynamic deadlift 1 x 15 Rower with barbell 1 x 15 Front squat 1 x 15 Front shoulder press 1 x 15 Repeat 3-5 times without stopping	Front squat 1 x 10 Rower with barbell 1 x 15 Walking lunge 1 x 5, each side Front shoulder press 1 x 15 Repeat 3-5 times without stopping
Cardio 5 min	Cardio 10 min
Note: The barbell must be the same light weight for all the exercises in the circuit. The subject will pick up the barbell at the start of the blitz and will not set it down until the end of the workout.	**Note:** The execution should not be too quick. It is important to find your own cadence and rhythm and to maintain it, improving gradually.

PROGRAM 3	PROGRAM 4
TONING	**ATHLETIC TRAINING**
Cardio 5 min: ideally walking, (stationary) steps, running, horizontal bike	Running or rope skipping 5 min
Squat 1 x 10 Front shoulder press 1 x 10 Walking lunge 1 x 10, each side Bar tractions (dips) 1 x 10 Repeat 5 times without stopping	Power swing (very heavy load) 1 x 10 Horizontal bench press 1 x 5 Power swing 1 x 10 Squat 1 x 5 Power swing 1 x 10 Chin-ups 1 x 5-7 Repeat 3-5 times without stopping
Cardio 5 min	Cardio 5 min
Note: Once you have grasped the blitz concept, it is important to move beyond these outlines and adapt them to our clients. Blitz circuits are extremely versatile and can be adapted to any subject, even beginners, by fine-tuning loads and intensity.	

PROGRAM 5	PROGRAM 6
FOR FEMALE SUBJECT WITH CELLULITE OR OTHER CIRCULATORY PROBLEMS	FOR MMA
Cardio 8 min	Rope skipping 8 min
Swing 1 x 10	Kettlebell clean and press 1 x 15
Push-up 1 x 10	Burpee 1 x 10
Front squat 1 x 5	Kettlebell squat and press 1 x 15
Rower with sandbag 1 x 10	Bar pull-up 1 x max
Step-up (two steps) 1 x 5, each side	Med ball lunge with rotation 1 x 10, each side
Repeat 3-5 times without stopping	Push-up 1 x 15
	Repeat 5-10 times without stopping
Cardio 8 min	
	Rope skipping 8 min
Note: The swing must be executed fast but with a rather light load. Load the front squat with 8 RM. The step-up exercise is essential to work on plantar arch circulation and help the venous blood flow.	**Note:** Plan a mini-recovery at the end of each circuit. Question: How long does a MMA bout last for? You will have to continue working non-stop on the circuit for the same amount of time. From here on, managing your energy levels throughout the bout will not be a problem.

PROGRAM 7	PROGRAM 8
GENERAL PHYSICAL PREPARATION	GENERAL PHYSICAL PREPARATION FOR WOMEN
Cardio 10 min	Cardio 10 min
Kettlebell squat and press 1 x 15	Kettlebell power swing 1 x 10
Sandbag snatch 1 x 10	At-the-shoulder sandbag squat 1 x 10, each side
Med ball diagonal press 1 x 10, each side	Floor pull 1 x 20
Crossover lunge 1 x 10, each side	One-leg kettlebell deadlift 1 x 10, each side
Rower with sandbag 1 x 20	Push-up 1 x 10
Side plank with twist 1 x 10, each side	Repeat 5-10 times without stopping
Repeat 5-10 times without stopping	
	Cardio 10 min
Cardio 10 min	

13.3.5   Timed circuits

The timed circuit concept was inspired by kettlebell work. In this type of circuit training you don't count sets and reps but only work for the preset time. You can apply this methodology, fine-tuning the exercises and the repetitions, on any type of subject: sedentary, intermediate, advanced, or athletes. You can also manage intensity (i.e., the effort expended in each single set), exercise by exercise, according to the student's degree of fitness and his or her special needs. Since the objective is long-duration work, managing the right level of intensity is clearly of utmost importance. For this reason I suggest starting with a load of about 10 RM, with only 5-6 reps per set.

PROGRAM 1	
ANTI-CELLULITE	
Uphill walking 15 min (3% slope; 2.8-3.1 mi/h [4.5-5 km/h]) Coreboard step-up 1 x 5, each leg Quadruped backward leg lift 1 x 10, each leg	Leg curl with fitness ball 1 x 5 Swing with kettlebell 1 x 10 Repeat for 10-20 min without stopping Uphill walking 15 min (3% slope; 2.5 mi/h [4 km/h])

Note: If the subject is a beginner, you will start with a 5-min workout, gradually increasing the time with each workout. Execution throughout the circuits will have to be extremely careful to maximize the training stimulus. The versatility of timed circuits and circuit training in general makes for virtually infinite combinations.

PROGRAM 2	
MULTI-DISTRICT WOMAN	
Uphill walking 10 min (3% slope; 2.8-3.1 mi/h [4.5-5 km/h]) Kettlebell or dumbbell swing 1 x 15 Quadruped backward leg lift 1 x 10, each leg Step-up on two steps 1 x 5, each leg Straight-leg quadruped lateral lunges 1 x 5, each leg Repeat for 10 min without stopping Cardio 5 min or active recovery 3 min Plank stabilization 1 x 20 sec Oblique crunches 1 x 5, each side	Lateral stabilization 1 x 15 sec, each side Reverse crunch 1 x 5 Repeat for 10 min without stopping Cardio 5 min Push press with dumbbells 1 x 6 Renegade row 1 x 5, each side Push-up 1 x 6 Floor pull 1 x 6 Repeat for 10 min without stopping Walking 10 min (cool-down)

PROGRAM 3	
TOTAL BODY	
Walking 10 min (warm-up)	Frontal stabilization 1 x 20 sec
Front squat 1 x 5	Repeat for 10 min without stopping
Floor pull 1 x 6	Cardio 5 min
Walking lunge 1 x 5, each leg	Kettlebell clean and press 1 x 6
Push press with kettlebell 1 x 6	Oblique rope crunches 1 x 10, each side
Repeat for 10 min without stopping	Swing with kettlebell 1 x 15
Cardio 5 min	Reverse rope crunch 1 x 10
Sandbag pull and press 1 x 6	Repeat for 10 min without stopping
Push-up 1 x 6	Walking (cool-down) 10 min
Rower with sandbag 1 x 6	

Note: Timed circuit training for advanced subjects marks the evolution from sportsperson to athlete; it forces you to refine your technique—your energy management and economy of gestures on the one hand and reduction of risks and increase in benefits on the other.

PROGRAM 4	
FOR THE INTERMEDIATE ATHLETE	
Run 10 min	At-the-shoulder sandbag lunge 1 x 6
Horizontal bench press 1 x 6	Med ball burpee 1 x 6
Front squat 1 x 6	Repeat for 10 min without stopping
Low pulley 1 x 6	Active recovery 3 min
One-leg kettlebell deadlift 1 x 5, each side	Kettlebell swing 1 x 10
Repeat for 10 min without stopping	Plyo push-up 1 x 5
Active recovery 3 min or cardio 5 min	Kettlebell deadlift 1 x 6
Kettlebell push press 1 x 6	Sandbag floor pull 1 x 6
Rower with sandbag 1 x 6	Repeat for 10 min without stopping
	Cardio 10 min

13.3.6   Boot camps

Boot camp training is a circuit training method based on the military courses used by soldiers worldwide for their operational training. It reached Italy, riding the popularity wave of training methods such as cross-fit and kettlebell training. It is an excellent, engaging group workout system. Boot camp training features a great variety in terms of exercise setting, exercise equipment, training intensity, and the management of groups ranging in numbers from 10 people to several hundreds. Boot camp training relies on the coach's ability in setting the course, planning the sequence and duration of exercises, and on the enthusiasm of fitness lovers ready to work out anywhere, whether in a park or a garage. I will never forget my experience at the summer 2012 boot camp in San Diego, California for the IDEA World Convention.

Warm-up: a 4 km (2.5 mi) run to the USS Midway aircraft carrier, moored in San Diego harbor. One hour of intense body-weight exercises led by Todd Durkin and his staff, then another 4-km cool-down run back to the San Diego Convention Center. Coming back to us, how can you set up a functional boot camp in a gym? This is actually rather simple. A lot depends on the number of people involved and the method used.

We shall therefore distinguish different approaches, based on a different number of stations according to how many the participants are. There are essentially three variables in this kind of circuit training:

1. the exercises
2. the exercise execution time
3. the recovery time between each station

The **exercises** must be extremely simple, especially for beginners and in each boot camp's initial circuits.

Execution time varies with each exercise. What does it depend on? On the objectives of the people you are training. Are you dealing with a group of athletes practicing lactacid or mixed sports (with energy delivery lasting from 30 sec and up)? Workout time will be 30-40 sec per station (as training progresses, you may increase this).

Are you dealing with a group of athletes practicing alactacid sports (power, expressions of strength, and explosiveness for 5-20 sec) ? Plan stations of 10-20 sec, up to a maximum of 30 sec. What about beginners, fitness lovers, and subjects with no competitive yearnings? Start with simple exercises lasting a maximum of 20 sec.

Moving from one station to another will be the circuit's active recovery time. This will have to be carefully measured out according to the subjects you are training. With athletes, the time can be progressively shortened, from 20 sec or less. You can actually turn the transfer from one station to another into an exercise; for example, you can reach the next station in a walking lunge, leopard plank, or leopard push-up. With beginners or occasional gym patrons, recovery time should definitely be higher. If the workout time at the station is, for example, 20 sec, recovery time between stations should be at least 30 sec. The last factor is space. The limit of an indoor boot camp is the space available. This is why I will restrict my indications to the number of people statistically more likely, given the usual size of gyms.

2 BOOT CAMP STATIONS
Groups between 8 and 20 people

Split the people into two distinct groups: Group 1 and Group 2. Group 1 (G1) will do a standing body-weight workout. Group 2 (G2) will work on mats. Assign an exercise to both groups. Execution time: Begin with 20 sec per station. Warm-up time: 10 min.

Circuit 1	Circuit 3
G1: squat 1 x 20 sec	G1: floor pull 1 x 20 sec
G2: crunch 1 x 20 sec	G2: reverse crunch 1 x 20 sec
Switch the exercises and repeat. Repeat this pair of exercises three times per group, with a 20-sec recovery time between exercises.	Switch the exercises and repeat. Repeat this pair of exercises three times per group, with a 20-sec recovery time between exercises.
Circuit 2	Circuit 4
G1: Walking lunge 1 x 20 sec	G1: leopard push-up
G2: arm stabilization 1 x 20 sec	G2: forearm stabilization 1 x 20 sec
Switch the exercises and repeat. Repeat this pair of exercises three times per group, with a 20-sec recovery time between exercises.	Switch the exercises and repeat. Repeat this pair of exercises three times per group, with a 20-sec recovery time between exercises.

4 BOOT CAMP STATIONS

Groups between 16 and 40 people

Split the participants into four groups:
G1, G2, G3, G4.
Set up four exercise stations: A, B, C, D.

Assign a muscle area to each station:

A = dynamic legs
B = core training
C = classic legs
D = trunk and upper body

Develop four exercises per station.

A
• Jumping jack
• Skip
• Starter
• Burpee

B
• Crunch
• Straight-arm plank
• Reverse crunch
• Plank with twist

C
• Squat
• Walking lunge
• Crab
• Lunge with rotation

D
• Push-up
• Lacerta push-up
• Leopard push-up
• Floor pull

Rules

1. Assign one group per station.

2. Assign and demonstrate to each group the first exercise in each station (Jumping jack, crunch, squat, push-up).

3. Start the clock: 20 sec to execute the maximum number of reps.

4. After 20 sec, stop the exercise and signal the station change.

5. Each group has 20 sec to transfer to the next exercise station.

6. Start the clock again for another 20 sec.

7. Repeat the sequence so that each group will complete the four stations circuit (Jumping jack, crunch, squat, push-up) three times.

8. Now pause so that athletes can recover and drink some water; then show each group the second exercise in each station (skip, straight-arm plank, walking lunge, lacerta push-up)

9. Start the cycle again, completing four circuits, with three sets per exercise.

ETHICS AND CONCLUSIONS

If you have come this far, then probably you are in it up to your neck... like me. Functional training improves your mind and body, makes you more open and observant, and, makes you a better person (why not?).

Your body will become a perfectly tailored outfit, your mind always lucid, and your senses focused to the max. You will enjoy your training and every moment of your life with an intensity you have never experienced before.

If you have come this far, please read these last few lines.

ETHICS OF THE FUNCTIONAL ATHLETE

1.   Train by using your body.

2.   Keep your eyes open, watch and discover new exercises.

3.   Always keep your mind open.

4.   Continue along your course: Improvement has no limits.

5.   Compare your method, you will find certainties.

6.   Love who you are and what you do.

Happy training, everybody!